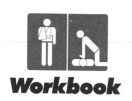

Workbook

American Red Cross
Standard First Aid

This participant's workbook is an integral part of the American Red Cross Standard First Aid course. By itself, it does not constitute adequate training for first aid. Please contact your Red Cross chapter for further information on this course.

ISBN: 0-86536-132-0

Acknowledgments

This course is based on the Standards and Guidelines established by the 1985 National Conference on Cardiopulmonary Resuscitation and Emergency Cardiac Care and on information provided by the Division of Medical Sciences, National Academy of Sciences, National Research Council.

This 1991 edition of the American Red Cross Standard First Aid workbook is designed to bring the 1989 edition to the current state of the art. These revisions also make Standard First Aid consistent with other Red Cross first aid courses. Several of those individuals who worked on the 1989 edition also contributed to this edition. The course and the original workbook are products of the 1987–1988 CPR/First Aid Project at the American Red Cross national headquarters. Units 2, 3, and 4 of the course are based on *American Red Cross: Adult CPR* (Stock No. 329128, © Feb. 1987).

Members of the American Red Cross Standard First Aid course design and development team were Karen J. Peterson, Ph.D.; Vikki Scott, M.P.A.; Zora Travis Salisbury, Ed.D.; Dennis L. Zaenger, M.P.H.; and Lawrence Newell, Ed.D. Assistance was provided by Program Development staff including: Bruce Spitz, Director; Frank Carrol; Jessica Bernstein, M.P.H.; Martha F. Beshers; Carol Hunter-Geboy, Ph.D.; Bryan MacNab Klinger; Pamela B. Mangu, M.A.; and Susan Walter.

The following national sector staff provided review and assistance: Charles R. Daniels; Joan E. Handler; Alfred J. Katz, M.D.; Carole Kauffman, R.N.; and John M. Malatak, M.S. Review was also provided by Red Cross chapter volunteers and staff: Mary M. "Posie" Mansfield; Joan S. Moiger, M.Ed.; Diana M. Meyer; and John Wagner.

Technical advice and review were provided by:
Allan Braslow, Ph.D., Faculty, 1985 National Conference on CPR and Emergency Cardiac Care; Braslow & Associates.

Frank P. Cooley, EMT-P, EMS Coordinator, Des Moines Fire Department, Des Moines, Iowa.

Rod Dennison, EMT-P, EMS Program Administrator, Texas Department of Health, Temple, Tex.

Stephan G. Lynn, M.D., FACEP, Director, Department of Emergency Medicine, St. Luke's/Roosevelt Hospital Center, New York, N.Y.

George E. Membrino, Ph.D., Associate Dean for Continuing Education and Associate Professor, Department of Family and Community Medicine, University of Massachusetts Medical School, Worcester, Mass.

William J. Schneiderman, Assistant Director, Medic IV Emergency Medical Services Project, Massachusetts Hospital Association, Burlington, Mass.

The manuscript was also reviewed by the National Academy of Sciences–National Research Council Committee to Advise the American National Red Cross; the Epilepsy Foundation of America; the American Diabetes Association, Inc.; and the National Capital Poison Center.

Field representatives providing advice and guidance through the 1987–1988 Red Cross First Aid Advisory Committee included:
Glenn Blafield, Greater Carolinas Chapter, Charlotte, N.C.

Bruce B. Bradley, AT&T Western United States, Sunnyvale, Calif.

Ruth Anne Chilldres, Tidewater Chapter, Virginia Beach Service Center, Norfolk, Va.

Wayne S. Doss, Springfield Chapter, Springfield, Mass.

Lori Jacob, St. Joseph County Chapter, South Bend, Ind.

Kevin Killeen, Southeastern Michigan Chapter, Detroit, Mich.

Nancy Kindelan, Los Angeles Chapter, Los Angeles, Calif.

David Lewis, Dallas Area Chapter, Dallas, Tex.

Robert T. Ogle, Madison County Chapter, Huntsville, Ala.

Gail Reebs, Western Operations Headquarters, Burlingame, Calif.

Dorothy E. Rust, Field Services, Minneapolis, Minn.

Lee Stapf, Midwestern Operations Headquarters, St. Louis, Mo.

Gary Sullivan, Mile High Chapter, Denver, Colo.

S. Corry Tanner, Salt Lake Area Chapter, Salt Lake City, Utah.

Angie Turner, R.N., Hawkeye Chapter, Waterloo, Iowa.

Barry White, Western Georgia Territory, Atlanta, Ga.

S. Elizabeth White, M.A.Ed., Actronics Corporation, Pittsburgh, Pa.

C. Stanley Williamson, Eastern Operations Headquarters, Alexandria, Va.

Acknowledgments

Red Cross chapters that participated in field tests included:
Greater Carolinas Chapter, Charlotte, N.C.
Madison County Chapter, Huntsville, Ala.
Northeast Georgia Chapter, Gainesville, Ga.
St. Croix Valley Chapter, Stillwater, Minn.
Salt Lake Area Chapter, Salt Lake, Utah
Santa Clara Valley Chapter, San Jose, Calif.
Southeastern Michigan Chapter, Detroit, Mich.

Groups participating in worksite field tests included:
Aetna Life Insurance Co., Charlotte, N.C.
AT&T Western United States, Sunnyvale, Calif.
City of Charlotte Engineering Department, Charlotte, N.C.
Detroit Edison Power Co., Detroit, Mich.
Ryder Rent-A-Truck, Romulus, Mich.

Contents

Contents

About This Course

As a person trained in first aid, you will join thousands of other people who are trained each year to save lives.

This course will prepare you to—
- Recognize the signs and symptoms of a heart attack.
- Help someone who is choking.
- Do the work of an unconscious person's heart and lungs until medical help arrives.
- Keep an injured person safe from further injury and as comfortable as possible until medical care can arrive.

Your family, friends, and fellow workers will also feel safer when they know that you have been trained by the American Red Cross in first aid.

By taking this course, you are showing your commitment to know what to do in an emergency. When you learn the information and skills presented in the course, you will be able to put your caring and concern for others into action.

Foundation of This First Aid Course

The American Red Cross believes that informed and trained citizens are the first link in the chain of those who help people in emergencies.

The Red Cross has been teaching first aid to the American public since the turn of this century, and **CPR (cardiopulmonary resuscitation)** since 1974. Over the years, the role of first aid has increased. One important development is the growth of **emergency medical services (EMS)** systems in most communities. Citizens trained in first aid need to know what to do before emergency medical services (EMS) arrives. This course recognizes that need. It integrates the lifesaving skills of **rescue breathing,** first aid for choking, and CPR with other essential but basic first aid skills.

This course has been designed to equip citizens to provide first aid to adult victims. While the principles in Section II in this course are generally applicable to children, the skills necessary to provide CPR to infants and children 1 through 8 years of age are taught in another course, American Red Cross CPR: Infant and Child. Parents and people working with young children are encouraged to take that course.

First Aid, CPR, and the Law

Legally, a victim must give consent to an offer to help before a person trained in first aid begins to help him or her. The law assumes that an unconscious person would give consent. If a victim is conscious, ask permission before helping him or her.

You should also make a reasonable attempt to get consent from the parent or guardian of a victim who is a minor or who is mentally or emotionally disturbed. If a parent or guardian is not available, you may give first aid without consent. Consent is also implied for a person who is unconscious, badly injured, or so ill that he or she cannot respond.

State "Good Samaritan" laws give legal protection to rescuers who act in good faith and are not guilty of gross negligence or willful misconduct. The type of rescuer covered and the scope of protection vary from state to state. Know your state's laws.

What You Will Learn

From this course you will learn how to provide first aid in emergencies. The skills and techniques you practice will—
• Help you to stay calm in emergencies because you know what to do.
• Help you to make decisions and take appropriate steps to keep a victim alive and keep injuries from becoming worse until EMS arrives.

These skills and techniques are presented in a way that teaches you both the rules and the important exceptions in first aid emergencies.

Every emergency requires you to follow first aid guidelines—the emergency action principles. You will learn to follow these emergency action principles to help find injuries and to take care of the most serious ones first.

Materials

Course materials have been developed to help you learn the basic concepts and skills necessary to give first aid.

Workbook
This workbook includes several features that make it an essential learning aid.

Each unit in the workbook begins with a list of objectives, which tell what you will learn in that unit.

The introductory material in each unit defines or describes specific medical emergencies; gives causes, signs, and symptoms of injuries; and explains appropriate first aid procedures.

Most units have an **action guide** that clearly and simply identifies the appropriate order of steps to take in giving first aid. This is a "how-to" guide for each major first aid topic.

Some units include skill sheets that give directions on how to perform certain first aid skills. You will be practicing these skills on a partner and/or on a **manikin.** By practicing some skills on a partner who will act as a victim, you will learn how it feels to work on a living person. For example, you will learn what a **pulse** actually feels like. Skill sheets will also indicate when you will have partner checks and instructor checks on your skill performance.

Videocassettes and Films
In some units you will see short videocassettes or films. These show situations in which you would use the skills learned in the course. They also contain demonstrations of the skills you will be practicing. Watching the demonstrations closely will help you do well in the practice sessions.

Tests

This course contains two types of tests: skill tests and written tests. Skill tests are given after you have practiced a skill and are ready to be tested by your instructor. A written test consisting of 25 questions is also given after each of the two sections of the course.

Certificates

Course completion certificates will be awarded to those participants who successfully complete the skill tests and pass the written tests with scores of 80 percent or better.

Activities

A variety of course activities has been designed to involve you more fully in the learning process. In addition to viewing the videocassettes or films, you will participate in the activities described below.

Practice on a Partner

When practicing on a partner, follow the checklist directions but do not make mouth-to-mouth contact; do not give actual rescue breaths; do not perform actual **chest compressions;** and do not perform actual **abdominal thrusts** or **chest thrusts.**

Practice on a Manikin

Before you start working on the manikin, clean the manikin's face and the inside of its mouth according to the directions given in this workbook on page xii.

Be sure the manikin's face and mouth have been cleaned before each member of your group practices, and also whenever you change places.

Partner Checks

When you are instructed to practice skills with a partner, have him or her read the skill sheet checklist out loud to you. It is important that you hear all the steps. The skill sheets not only help you learn the steps in the correct order but also give you information about the victim's condition.

You will practice until you can perform the skills correctly, confidently, and in the right order, without having your partner read the directions to you.

When you can perform the skills correctly without coaching from your partner, he or she will watch you go through the whole procedure, checking off each step in the "Partner Check" column on the skill sheets as you do it. After your partner has checked you, clean the manikin, change places, and go through the same procedure while he or she practices.

If you need help during the practice session, ask your instructor to help you, or refer to this workbook.

About This Course

Instructor Checks

The instructor will check your skills by having you go through the whole procedure without prompting. If the instructor sees a serious error, he or she will stop checking and correct you. You will then practice the skill correctly. When you feel you are ready to be checked again, ask the instructor to recheck you. After you have completed the entire procedure correctly, the instructor will sign your workbook.

Some Health Precautions and Guidelines

You may be concerned about the possibility of contracting an infectious disease when you provide basic first aid. The following information addresses some of the most common health concerns in providing first aid and in using the equipment in this class.

First Aid and Infectious Diseases

You will probably use your first aid skills to help someone whom you know personally—a family member, a friend, a co-worker. For this reason it is possible you will know your risk of contracting an **infectious disease.** As a person trained in first aid, you should know that there are **blood-borne** diseases such as hepatitis and HIV (the AIDS virus) and **air-borne** diseases such as influenza. Adopt practices that discourage the spread of disease when performing first aid.

Although it does not often happen, several blood-borne infectious diseases can be transmitted through direct contact between the blood of an infected person and sores or open cuts on your skin or in your mouth. To reduce the risk of being infected when you attempt to control bleeding, use some sort of barrier, such as several dressings, latex gloves, or a piece of plastic wrap, between you and the victim's blood if possible. Wearing latex gloves helps you to avoid direct skin contact with other body fluids such as vomit, feces, or urine. Always wash your hands as soon as you can after giving first aid.

Some air-borne infectious diseases and viruses can be transmitted by the air we breathe. A person trained in first aid exchanges air with a victim during rescue breathing. You will probably know the person on whom you will perform rescue breathing; therefore you may know the likelihood of contracting an infectious disease or virus from that person's breath.

Saliva exchange during mouth-to-mouth contact is another method of possible infectious disease transmission. Rescue breathing and CPR generally involve mouth-to-mouth contact. A person trained in first aid may risk contracting some viruses and infectious diseases from saliva in order to save a life. However, at the writing date of this manual, there is no evidence that you can be infected by hepatitis B virus or HIV (AIDS virus) either through contact with human saliva or by giving rescue breathing.

CPR Training and Infectious Diseases

Since the beginning of citizen training in CPR (cardiopulmonary resuscitation), the American Red Cross and the American Heart Association have trained more than 50 million people in these lifesaving skills. According to the Centers for Disease Control (CDC), there has never been a documented case of any infectious disease transmitted through the use of CPR manikins.

The Red Cross follows widely accepted guidelines for the cleaning and decontamination of training manikins. **If these guidelines are consistently followed, and basic personal hygiene (for example, frequent handwashing) is practiced, the risk of any kind of disease transmission during CPR training is extremely low.**

There are also some **health precautions** and guidelines that you should know. You should take these precautions if you have an acute or chronic infection or have a condition that would increase your risk or the other participants' risk of exposure to infections. Most acute infections or conditions, such as a cold, a cut on the hand, or breaks in the skin in or around the mouth, are short-lived. The safest and most practical thing to do if you have an acute infection or condition is to postpone CPR training until, for instance, your cut or abrasion heals, or your cold or influenza is over.

Other infections and conditions may be chronic, or require a longer recovery period, making it impractical to postpone CPR training. In this instance, for your safety and the safety of others, it may be appropriate for you to use a separate manikin for CPR training, after you have discussed your participation with your private physician.

You should **postpone** participation in CPR training if you—
- Have a respiratory infection, such as a cold or a sore throat.
- Believe or know you have recently been exposed to any infection, to which you may be susceptible.
- Are showing signs and symptoms of any infectious disease such as a cold, chicken pox, or mumps, or if you have a fever.
- Have any cuts or sores on your hands, or in or around your mouth (for example, cold sores or recent tooth extraction).
- Know you are seropositive (have had a positive blood test) for hepatitis B surface antigen (HBsAg), indicating that you are currently infected with hepatitis B virus.*

You should request a **separate manikin** if you—
- Know you have a chronic infection such as indicated by long-term seropositivity (long-term positive blood tests) for hepatitis B surface antigen (HBsAg)* or a positive test for anti-HIV (that is, a positive test for antibodies to HIV, the virus that causes AIDS).
- Have an acute infection or condition but are unable to postpone CPR training.
- Have a type of condition that makes you unusually susceptible to infection.

If, after you read and consider the above information, you decide that you need to have your own manikin, ask your instructor if one can be made available for your use. If you qualify under the above conditions for the use of a separate manikin, you should discuss this with your instructor, but you will not be required to provide details in your request. The manikin will not be used by anyone else until it has been cleaned according to the recommended end-of-class decontamination procedures. The Red Cross will do its best to provide you with a separate manikin. However, please understand that it may be impossible to do so, especially on short notice, because of limited numbers of manikins for class use. In this instance, you may wish to reschedule CPR training for a later date. The more advance notice you provide, the more likely it is that the Red Cross will be able to accommodate your request.

Guidelines to Follow During Training

To protect yourself and other participants from infection, you should do the following:
- Wash your hands thoroughly before working with the manikin and repeat handwashing as often as is necessary or appropriate.
- Do not eat, drink, use tobacco products, or chew gum immediately before or during manikin use.
- Before you use the manikin, dry the manikin's face with a clean gauze pad. Next, vigorously wipe the manikin's face and the inside of its mouth with a clean gauze pad soaked with either a solution of liquid chlorine bleach and water (sodium hypochlorite and water) or rubbing alcohol. Place this wet pad over the manikin's mouth and nose and wait at least 30 seconds. Then wipe the face dry with a clean gauze pad.
- When practicing what to do for an obstructed airway, simulate (pretend to do) the finger sweep.

Physical Stress and Injury

CPR requires strenuous activity. If you have a medical condition or disability that will prevent you from taking part in the practice sessions, please let your instructor know.

Damage to Manikins

In order to protect the manikins from damage, you should do the following before you begin to practice:
- Remove pens and pencils from your pockets.
- Remove all jewelry.
- Remove lipstick and excess makeup.
- Remove chewing gum and candy from your mouth.

---

*A person with hepatitis B infection will test positive for the hepatitis B surface antigen (HBsAg). Most persons infected with hepatitis B will get better within a period of time. However, some hepatitis B infections will become chronic and will linger for much longer. These persons will continue to test positive for HBsAg, and their decision to participate in CPR training should be guided by their physician.

After a person has had an acute hepatitis B infection, he or she will no longer test positive for the surface antigen but will test positive for the hepatitis B antibody (anti-HBs). Persons who have been vaccinated for hepatitis B will also test positive for the hepatitis antibody. A positive test for the hepatitis B antibody (anti-HBs) should not be confused with a positive test for the hepatitis B surface antigen (HBsAg).

Section I

1 Emergency Action Principles

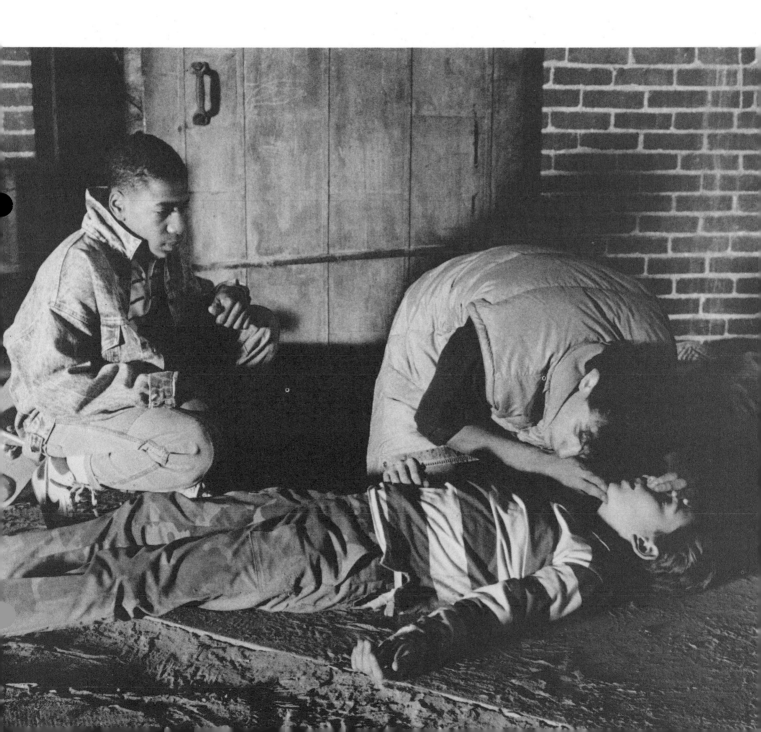

Emergency Action Principles

Learning Objectives

In this unit you will learn how to—
1. Survey the scene.
2. Do a primary survey of the victim.
3. Phone the emergency medical services (EMS) system for help.
4. Do a secondary survey of the victim.

Developing first aid common sense is an important part of providing first aid care. First aid, properly given, can reduce the effects of injuries and medical emergencies, can keep a seriously ill or injured person alive, and can mean the difference between a short and a long hospital stay. Proper first aid must be given quickly and effectively or the victim's condition may become more serious by the time further help arrives on the scene.

In the excitement of an emergency, it is important to stop for a moment to clear your head and think before you act. When responding to an emergency situation, remain calm and apply the four emergency action principles:

1. Survey the scene.
2. Do a primary survey of the victim.
3. Phone the emergency medical services (EMS) system for help.
4. Do a secondary survey of the victim, when appropriate.

Survey the Scene

When you respond in an emergency, make a quick, decision-making survey of the entire scene. Don't look only at the victim; look at the area around the victim. This should take only a few seconds. Decide what needs to be done immediately and the order in which you will take other steps. Consider the following as you do your survey:

1. Is the scene safe?

You must first decide if the situation is safe for you. You cannot help the victim by becoming a victim yourself. Know your abilities. If you cannot get to the victim because of extreme hazards, such as fire, toxic fumes, heavy traffic, electrical wires, or deep or swift-moving water, call EMS. In addition to sending medical care, the EMS dispatcher can contact the fire department, police department, park rangers, lifeguards, power company, or other services needed to handle the specific life-threatening hazard.

If you can safely get to the victim, decide if it is safe to remain at the scene while you continue the steps of the emergency action principles and care for the victim. If it is not safe, you may need to make an immediate emergency rescue. As a general rule, however, do not move an injured person if you do not have to.

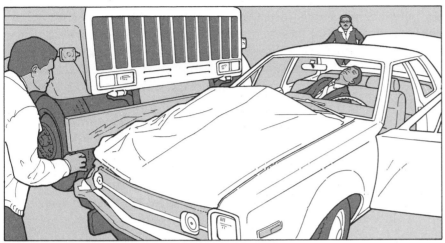

Figure 1
Survey the Scene

2. What happened?

If the victim is conscious, ask specific questions to determine what happened and the extent of the victim's illness or injury. If the victim is unconscious and you are unable to determine what caused the illness or injury, then look around for clues. The scene itself often gives the answers *(Fig. 1)*.

If a person is lying next to a ladder, you may suspect that he or she fell off the ladder and may have broken bones and bruises. An electrical wire on the ground at the scene may mean that the victim has suffered an electric shock. This kind of information is important, especially when the victim is unconscious and cannot tell you what is wrong.

Quickly look for a **medical alert tag** at the neck or wrist. If the victim is not responsive, this tag may provide some information about what might be wrong and how you should care for him or her.

Some accidents may cause head, neck, or back injuries that, if not treated properly, could lead to permanent paralysis or even death. Any victim who complains of pain in the head, neck, or back, or is found unconscious after an accident, must be cared for as if he or she has a spinal (neck or back) injury. At the scene of this type of injury, you might find clues such as a car with a shattered windshield, scaffolding that has collapsed, cuts, bleeding from the ears or nose, or bruises on the victim's head, neck, or face that are indicators of possible spinal injuries.

3. How many people are injured?

Look beyond the victim you see at first glance. There may be other victims. One person may be screaming while another, who may be more seriously injured or unconscious, is unnoticed. In an auto accident, car doors that are open may mean there are more victims nearby who were thrown from or walked away from the car.

4. Are there bystanders who can help?
If there are bystanders, use them to help you find out what happened. If anyone knows the victim, ask if the victim has any medical problems. This information can help you determine what may be wrong. Bystanders, although they may not be trained in first aid, can help you in other important ways, such as by calling EMS; by offering emotional support to the victims, their friends, and their families; and by keeping onlookers from getting too close to the scene.

Identify Yourself as a Person Trained in First Aid
Tell the victim and bystanders who you are and that you are trained in first aid. This may help to reassure the victim. It will also help you take charge of the situation, letting others who may have been caring for the victim know that a trained person is on hand.

Before giving first aid to a conscious victim, it is important that you obtain his or her consent. Consent should be obtained from all mentally competent, conscious adults. Asking for consent is a matter of a simple question. Say, "Hi, my name is _____. I know first aid and I can help you until an ambulance arrives; is that OK?" For minors and mentally or emotionally disturbed victims, make a reasonable attempt to get permission from a parent or legal guardian. If a parent or guardian is not available, first aid care may be given without consent. If a victim is unconscious, badly injured, or so ill that he or she cannot respond, consent is implied. The law assumes that consent would have been given.

Do a Primary Survey of the Victim

The purpose of a primary survey is to check for life-threatening conditions and to give urgent first aid care.

When you come upon the scene of an accident that you did not witness, you may find a victim who is not moving. You must determine whether the victim is conscious and responsive or is unconscious. You can generally tell if the person is responsive by gently tapping the person on the shoulder and asking, "Are you OK?"

Some injuries or illnesses may require assistance in caring for the victim or calling EMS. If this is the case, you may need to shout several times to get someone's attention. While you are seeking help, continue the primary survey by checking for an open **airway**, breathing, and circulation (**pulse** and severe bleeding). This is known as checking the **ABCs:**

Check the Airway

Does the victim have an open airway (the passage that allows the victim to breathe)? The most important action for successful **resuscitation** is to immediately open an unconscious victim's airway using the head-tilt/chin-lift method *(Fig. 2).* It lifts the tongue away from the back of the throat and opens the airway. Detailed steps are given in skill sheets (page 19). (Some people breathe through an opening in the front of the neck called a stoma. See page 24.)

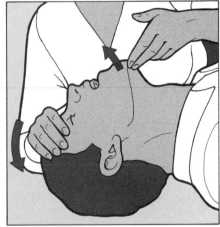

Figure 2
Head-tilt/Chin-lift

Check Breathing

Check for **breathlessness.** (Is the person breathing?) Look for the chest to rise and fall, listen for breathing, and feel for air coming out of the victim's nose and mouth *(Fig. 3).*

If the victim is breathing, you will see chest movement and hear and feel escaping air at your ear and cheek. Chest movement alone does not mean that the victim is breathing. If the victim is not breathing, you must give two full breaths to get air into the lungs. If the victim has a pulse but is not breathing, you will need to breathe for him or her. This is called rescue breathing (see Unit 2).

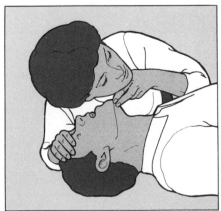

Figure 3
Check for Breathlessness

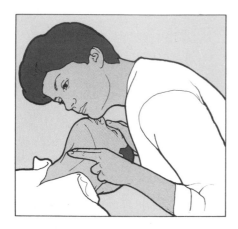

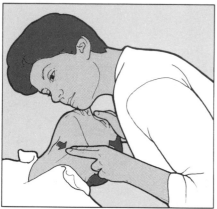

Figure 4
Locate and Feel Carotid Pulse

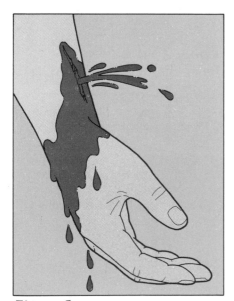

Figure 5a
Severe Bleeding

**Check
Circulation**

1. Is the person's heart beating? If a person is breathing, his or her heart is beating and is circulating blood. If the person is not breathing, you must find out if the heart is beating. You do this by checking his or her pulse. Feel for a pulse at the side of the neck. This pulse is called the **carotid pulse** *(Fig. 4)*. Detailed steps for checking the carotid pulse are given in the rescue breathing skill sheets (page 20). If the person does not have a pulse, you will need to give **cardiopulmonary resuscitation (CPR)** to keep oxygen-rich blood circulating (see Unit 4).

2. Is the person bleeding severely? To check for bleeding, look over the victim's body quickly for wet, blood-soaked clothing. Bleeding is severe when blood spurts from the wound (arterial bleeding) or cannot be controlled *(Fig. 5a)*. Check for severe bleeding by looking from head to toe for signs of external bleeding *(Fig. 5b)*. First check the pulse, then control any severe bleeding.

Complete the primary survey before actually giving any urgent first aid. Life-threatening conditions must be cared for before less serious conditions. It is more important, for example, to give rescue breathing to someone who is not breathing than to splint a broken arm or bandage a small cut.

If no one has responded to your shouts for help by the end of one minute of giving urgent first aid, you should get to a phone as quickly as you can and phone EMS. Then quickly return to the victim and continue first aid.

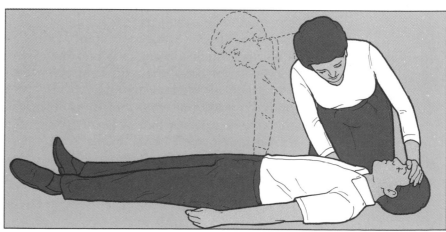

Figure 5b
Check for Severe Bleeding

Phone the Emergency Medical Services (EMS) System for Help

An emergency medical services (EMS) system is a community-wide, coordinated means of responding to an accident or a medical emergency. As a person trained in first aid, you are the first link in your community's emergency response chain. When you come upon the scene of an injury or sudden illness, and after you have completed a primary survey, you can activate a professional system that provides advanced care and skilled transfer of the victim to a medical facility.

EMS should be activated for life-threatening conditions that require the assistance of trained medical professionals. As a general rule, call EMS personnel if any of the following conditions exist:
- Unconsciousness or altered level of consciousness
- Breathing problems (difficulty breathing or no breathing)
- Persistent chest or abdominal pain or pressure
- No pulse
- Severe bleeding
- Vomiting blood or passing blood
- Poisoning
- Seizures, severe headache, or slurred speech
- Injuries to head, neck, or back
- Possible broken bones

There are also special situations that warrant calling EMS personnel for assistance. These include—
- Fire or explosion.
- The presence of poisonous gas.
- Downed electrical wires.
- Swift-moving water.
- Motor vehicle collisions.
- Victims who cannot be moved easily.

There may be times when you as a person trained in basic first aid will be providing care to someone with a minor injury such as a skinned elbow, nosebleed, or broken finger. In minor situations such as these, it may not be necessary to phone EMS since you may be able to care for the minor wound or transport the individual to a medical facility yourself. Common sense and prudent behavior will guide you in making the right decision. But remember, if in doubt phone EMS for help. Using what you learn in this course will help you decide when it is necessary to call EMS.

Prehospital EMS care provides an arm of the hospital emergency room that extends into the community. EMS teams will respond quickly with the knowledge and the necessary equipment to rescue, stabilize, and transport victims.

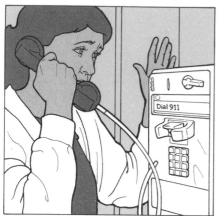

Figure 6
Phone the EMS System

Many communities have a 9-1-1 emergency number telephone system to activate the EMS team. By dialing 9-1-1, people in the community can activate an ambulance service, the police department, and the fire department. Some communities have a local number to call for an ambulance; in others, the operator forwards emergency calls. Be sure to know what number to use in your community.

Making the Call

Make the call to EMS yourself, or give that responsibility to bystanders *(Fig. 6)*. If possible, send two people to make the call, to ensure it is made accurately. Instruct the caller(s) to report back to you and tell you what the dispatcher said.

It is very important to stay on the phone after you have given all of the information listed below in case the **EMS dispatcher** has any further questions. Make sure that the dispatcher has all the information to get the right help to the scene quickly. Be prepared to tell the dispatcher—

• The location of the emergency (exact address, city or town, nearby intersections, landmarks, name of building, floor, apartment or room number).
• The telephone number of the phone being used.
• The caller's name.
• What happened.
• The number of victims.
• The victims' conditions.
• The help being given.

Remember—do not hang up first, because the dispatcher may need more information. For a more detailed description of the EMS System, see the Appendix.

Do a Secondary Survey of the Victim

The purpose of a secondary survey is to check the victim carefully and in an orderly way for injuries or other problems that are not an immediate threat to life but which could cause problems if not corrected. For example, a secondary survey may lead you to suspect that the victim has a broken bone. This may not be immediately life-threatening but could become a serious problem if ignored. The steps of a secondary survey are to interview the victim and bystanders; check the **vital signs** (pulse, breathing, and skin appearance and temperature); and do a head-to-toe exam. The detailed steps of the secondary survey are covered in Section II of this course.

The Emergency Action Principles Action Guide provides you with an overview of what you will learn in this course.

Deciding to Transport the Victim

After completing the EAPs, you might consider transporting the victim to the hospital yourself if the victim's condition is not severe. This is an important decision. Do not transport a victim with a life-threatening condition or one in whom there is any chance that a life-threatening condition may develop. In these instances, call EMS personnel and wait for help. A car trip can be painful for the victim, and may aggravate the injury or cause additional injury.

If you do decide to transport the victim yourself, ask someone else to come with you. One person should drive while the other helps keep the victim comfortable. Be sure you know the quickest route to the nearest medical facility with emergency care capabilities. Pay close attention to the victim, and watch for any changes in his or her condition.

Discourage a victim from driving to the hospital. An injury may restrict movement, or the victim may become groggy or faint. A sudden onset of pain may be distracting. Also, an injured or ill person may drive faster than he or she would normally. Any of these conditions can make driving dangerous for the victim, passengers, pedestrians, and other drivers.

There may be some situations, however, when an ambulance is not readily available, and you may have to weigh the risks and consider driving the victim to the hospital. You should know that not all hospitals and health facilities offer advanced care, and of those that do, not all offer it on a 24-hour basis. Therefore, it is important to be familiar with the emergency resources of your community and develop a plan of action before an emergency happens.

Emergency Action Principles Action Guide

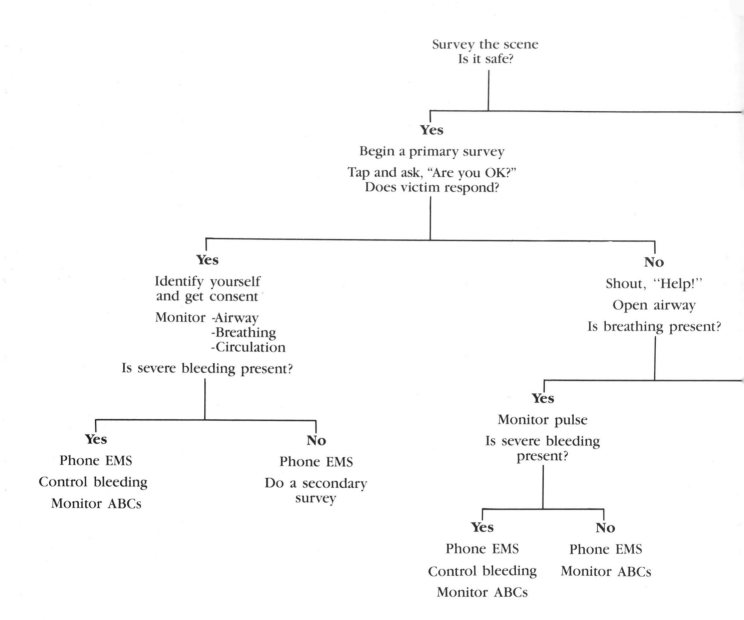

Survey the scene
Is it safe?

Yes

Begin a primary survey

Tap and ask, "Are you OK?"
Does victim respond?

Yes

Identify yourself
and get consent

Monitor -Airway
-Breathing
-Circulation

Is severe bleeding present?

Yes
Phone EMS
Control bleeding
Monitor ABCs

No
Phone EMS
Do a secondary
survey

No

Shout, "Help!"
Open airway
Is breathing present?

Yes

Monitor pulse
Is severe bleeding
present?

Yes
Phone EMS
Control bleeding
Monitor ABCs

No
Phone EMS
Monitor ABCs

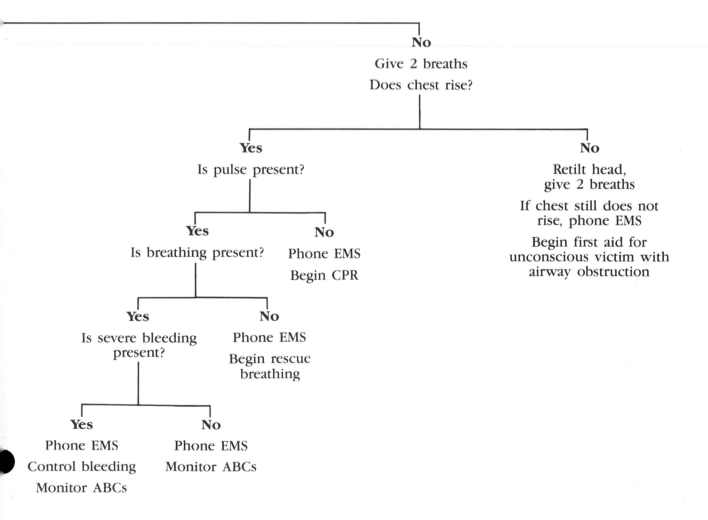

No
Phone EMS
Stay clear of danger

No
Give 2 breaths
Does chest rise?

Yes
Is pulse present?

No
Retilt head,
give 2 breaths

If chest still does not
rise, phone EMS

Begin first aid for
unconscious victim with
airway obstruction

Yes
Is breathing present?

No
Phone EMS
Begin CPR

Yes
Is severe bleeding
present?

No
Phone EMS
Begin rescue
breathing

Yes
Phone EMS
Control bleeding
Monitor ABCs

No
Phone EMS
Monitor ABCs

2   *Rescue Breathing*

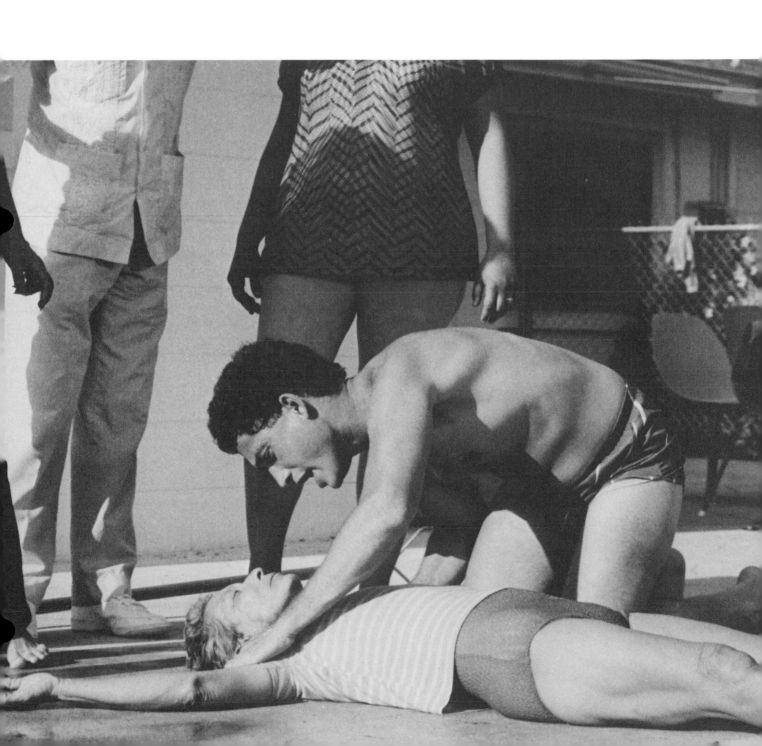

Rescue Breathing

Learning Objectives

In this unit you will learn how to—
1. *Recognize a breathing emergency.*
2. *Position a victim for rescue breathing.*
3. *Perform rescue breathing.*

Definition

Rescue breathing is a way of breathing air into someone's lungs when natural breathing has stopped or a person cannot breathe properly on his or her own. This is also known as **artificial respiration.**

Respiratory and Circulatory Systems

When we breathe in, air enters the body through the nose and mouth. It travels down the throat, through the windpipe, and into the lungs. These body parts make up our breathing, or **respiratory system.** The pathway from the nose and mouth to the lungs is called the airway. For air to enter the lungs, the airway must be open. Air contains **oxygen,** which the body needs to live. In the lungs the oxygen in the air is transferred to the blood. The **oxygen-rich blood** is then carried throughout the body by the **circulatory system.**

If either the respiratory or the circulatory system fails to function properly, the supply of oxygen to the body is decreased and the person may soon die. In such cases the victim needs rescue breathing (or CPR if the heart stops) to stay alive until EMS arrives. Without a constant supply of oxygen, the brain will begin to die within four to six minutes. Rescue breathing works because the air you breathe into the victim contains more than enough oxygen to keep that person alive. The air you take in with every breath is about 21 percent oxygen, but your body uses only a small part of that. The air you breathe out of your own lungs and into the lungs of the victim is about 16 percent oxygen, enough oxygen to keep someone alive.

Common Causes of Breathing Emergencies

Breathing emergencies may be caused by—
* **Airway obstructions.**
* Poisonous substances.
* Injury to the chest or lungs.
* Near-drowning.
* Electrocution.
* Certain drugs.
* Burns.
* Certain diseases and illnesses.
* Reactions to insect bites and stings.
* Shock.

The Technique

To find out if a person needs rescue breathing, begin with a primary survey to check the ABCs:
1. Check for **unresponsiveness.**
2. If no response, shout, "Help!"
3. Position the victim on his or her back.
4. Open the airway
5. Look, listen, and feel for breathing.
6. If the person is not breathing, give 2 full breaths.
7. Check the carotid pulse and check for severe bleeding.
8. Have someone phone EMS for help.

If the victim is not breathing but has a pulse, begin rescue breathing. To give rescue breathing keep the airway open with the head-tilt/chin-lift. Then give one breath every 5 seconds. Each breath should last 1 to 1½ seconds. After one minute recheck the carotid pulse. Then continue giving one breath every 5 seconds. These steps keep air flowing to the victim's lungs.

Refer to the skill sheets for the step-by-step procedure for giving rescue breathing.

A Commonly Asked Question About Rescue Breathing

1. Q. Can a person be breathing and not have a pulse?
   A. No. When the heart stops beating, blood no longer circulates through the body, which deprives the cells of oxygen. This causes the respiratory system to shut down and the person to stop breathing.

Skill Sheets: Rescue Breathing

You find a person lying on the ground, not moving. First survey the scene to see if it is safe, and to get some idea of what has happened. Then do a primary survey by checking for unresponsiveness, then checking the ABCs.

Note: Before you practice on a manikin, clean its face and the inside of its mouth. Follow the directions on page xii. Clean the manikin's face and mouth before each person practices.

   Check for Unresponsiveness (Does victim respond?)

Tap or gently shake victim.

Ask, "Are you OK?"

If no response: Shout, "Help!"

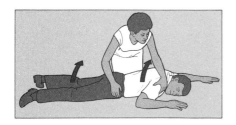

□ □   **Position the Victim**

Roll victim onto back, if necessary.

Kneel facing victim, midway between victim's hips and shoulders.

Straighten victim's legs, if necessary, and move arm closer to you above victim's head.

Lean over victim, and place one hand on victim's shoulder and other hand on victim's hip.

Roll victim toward you as a single unit; as you roll victim, move your hand from shoulder to support back of head and neck.

Place victim's arm nearer you alongside victim's body.

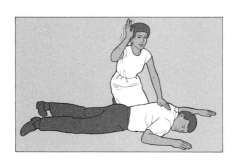

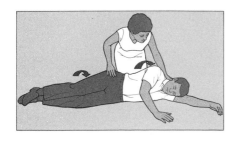

Partner Check
Instructor Check

☐ ☐ **Open the Airway** (Use head-tilt/chin-lift method)

Place your hand—the one nearer victim's head—on victim's forehead.

Place 2 fingers of other hand under bony part of lower jaw near chin.

Tilt head and lift jaw. Avoid closing victim's mouth. Avoid pushing on soft parts under chin.

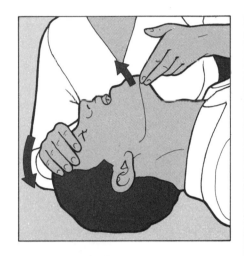

☐ ☐ **Check for Breathlessness** (Is victim breathing?)

Maintain open airway.

Place your ear over victim's mouth and nose.

Look at chest, listen, and feel for breathing for 3 to 5 seconds.

Say, "No breathing."

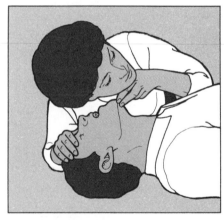

☐ ☐ **Give 2 Full Breaths**

Maintain open airway.

Pinch nose shut.

Open your mouth wide, take a deep breath, and make a tight seal around outside of victim's mouth.

Give 2 full breaths. Each breath should last 1 to 1½ seconds. Pause between each breath for you to take a breath.

Look for chest to rise and fall. Listen and feel for escaping air.

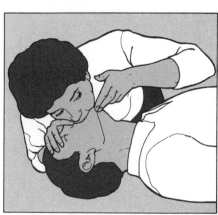

Partner Check
Instructor Check

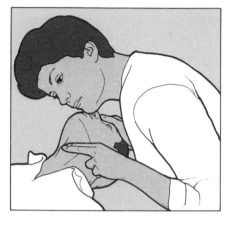

☐ ☐ **Check for Carotid Pulse**

Maintain head-tilt with one hand on victim's forehead.

Locate **Adam's apple** with middle and index fingers of other hand.

Slide fingers down into groove of neck on side closer to you.

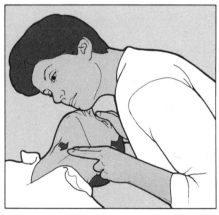

Feel for carotid pulse for 5 to 10 seconds.

Say, "No breathing, but there is a pulse."

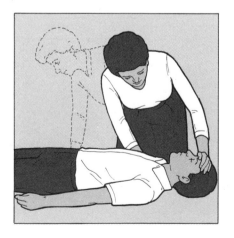

☐ ☐ **Check for Severe Bleeding**

Look over the victim's body quickly to see if he or she is bleeding severely.

☐ ☐ **Phone EMS for Help**

Tell someone to call for an ambulance.

Say, "No breathing, has a pulse, call _____" (Local emergency number or Operator).

☐ ☐ **Begin Rescue Breathing**

Maintain open airway with head-tilt/chin-lift.

Pinch nose shut.

Open your mouth wide, take a deep breath, and make a tight seal around outside of victim's mouth.

Give 1 breath every 5 seconds. Each breath should last 1 to 1½ seconds. Count aloud "one one-thousand, two one-thousand, three one-thousand, four one-thousand," take a breath yourself, and then give a breath.

Look for the chest to rise and fall. Listen and feel for escaping air and return of breathing. Continue for 1 minute—about 12 breaths.

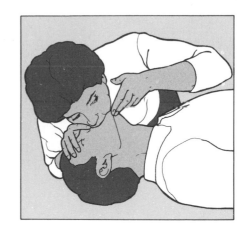

☐ ☐ **Recheck Carotid Pulse**

Maintain head-tilt with one hand on victim's forehead.

Locate carotid pulse and feel for 5 seconds.

Say, "Has pulse."

Next look, listen, and feel for breathing for 3 to 5 seconds.

Say, "No breathing."

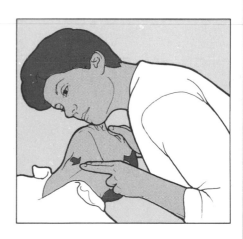

Rescue Breathing Skill Sheets

☐ ☐ **Continue Rescue Breathing**

Maintain open airway with head-tilt/chin-lift.

Give 1 breath every 5 seconds. Each breath should last 1 to 1½ seconds.

Recheck pulse every minute.

☐ ☐ **What To Do Next**

If pulse is absent, begin CPR.

If pulse is present but victim still not breathing, continue rescue breathing.

If victim begins to breathe, maintain open airway, and monitor breathing until EMS arrives.

Final Instructor Check _____

Special Situations

Air in the Stomach (Gastric Distention)

While doing rescue breathing, be careful not to breathe air into the victim's stomach. Air in the stomach can be a serious problem. It can cause the victim to vomit. When an unconscious person vomits, the stomach contents may go into the lungs. That can lead to death.

During rescue breathing, air can enter the stomach in three ways:

- Breathing into the victim after the chest has risen. This causes extra air to fill the stomach.
- Not tilting the victim's head back far enough to open the airway completely and then breathing at greater pressure to fill the victim's lungs.
- Giving breaths too quickly. Quick breaths are given with higher pressure, which causes air to enter the stomach.

To avoid forcing air into the stomach, make sure you keep the victim's head tilted all the way back. Breathe into the victim only enough to make the chest rise. Don't give breaths too quickly; pause between breaths long enough to let the victim's lungs empty and for you to get another breath.

If you notice that the victim's stomach has begun to bulge, make sure that the head is tilted back far enough and make sure you are not breathing into the victim too hard or too fast.

Vomiting

Sometimes while you are helping an unconscious victim, the victim may vomit. If this happens, turn the victim's head and body to one side, quickly wipe the material out of the victim's mouth, and continue where you left off.

Mouth-to-Nose Breathing

Use the **mouth-to-nose breathing** method when the victim's mouth or jaw is injured, the victim is bleeding from the mouth, the jaw cannot be opened, or if your mouth is too small to make a tight seal. Mouth-to-nose breathing should be done as follows:

- Maintain the backward head-tilt position with one hand on the forehead. Use the other hand to close the mouth and lift the chin.
- Open your mouth wide, take a deep breath, seal your mouth tightly around the victim's nose, and breathe full breaths into the victim's nose *(Fig. 7)*, as described for the mouth-to-mouth method in the skill sheets. Open the victim's mouth between breaths, if possible, to allow air to come out.

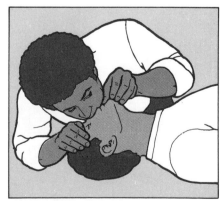

Figure 7
Mouth-to-Nose Breathing

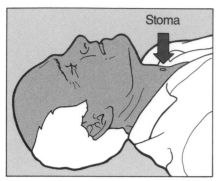

Figure 8
Victim With a Stoma

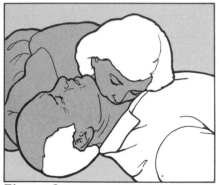

Figure 9
Mouth-to-Stoma Breathing

Mouth-to-Stoma Breathing

There are some people who have had surgery to remove all or part of the upper end of the windpipe. They breathe through an opening called a **stoma** in the front of the neck *(Fig. 8)*. This takes the air right into the windpipe, bypassing both the mouth and nose.

To give rescue breathing to someone with a stoma, you must give breaths through the stoma and not through the mouth or nose. In **mouth-to-stoma breathing,** you follow the same basic steps as in the mouth-to-mouth method, except that you:

1. Look, listen, and feel for breathing with your ear held over the stoma.
2. Give breaths into the stoma, breathing at the same rate as for mouth-to-mouth breathing *(Fig. 9)*.

There are several other important things you should remember when you give rescue breathing to someone who breathes through a stoma:

- Don't tilt the victim's head back.
- Don't breathe air into the victim through his or her nose or mouth. This may fill the victim's stomach with air.
- Never block the stoma, since it is the only way the victim has to breathe.
- In some instances a person who has had only part of the upper end of his or her windpipe removed may breathe through the stoma as well as the nose and mouth. If the person's chest does not rise when you breathe through the stoma, you should close off the mouth and nose and continue breathing through the stoma.

Victims With Dentures

If a victim who needs rescue breathing is wearing dentures, leave the dentures in place if they have not moved. They will give support to the mouth and cheeks during mouth-to-mouth breathing. Even if the dentures are loose, the head-tilt/chin-lift described earlier may help keep them in place. If the dentures become so loose that they block the airway or make it difficult for you to give breaths, take them out.

When Head, Neck, or Back (Spinal) Injuries Are Suspected

Most conditions requiring rescue breathing (or CPR) are not due to or associated with major injuries. However, head, neck, or back injuries should be suspected if victims were subjected to a violent force, such as that which results from a motor vehicle crash or a fall. If you suspect the victim may have an injury to the head, neck, or back, you should try to minimize movement of the head and neck when opening the airway. This requires you to modify the head-tilt/chin-lift.

First try to open the victim's airway by lifting the chin without tilting the head back *(Fig. 10)*. This may be enough to allow air to pass into the lungs. If you attempt rescue breathing and your breaths are not going in, you should tilt the head back very slightly. In most cases, this will be enough to allow air to pass into the lungs. If air still does not go in, tilt the head further back. It is unlikely that this action will cause any additional injury to the victim. A person who is not breathing needs oxygen. Therefore, opening the airway is the primary concern.

Additional methods for handling these victims are discussed in the American Red Cross CPR: Basic Life Support for the Professional Rescuer course.

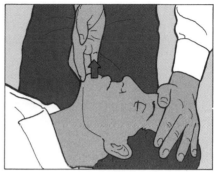

Figure 10
Chin Lift

Rescue Breathing Action Guide

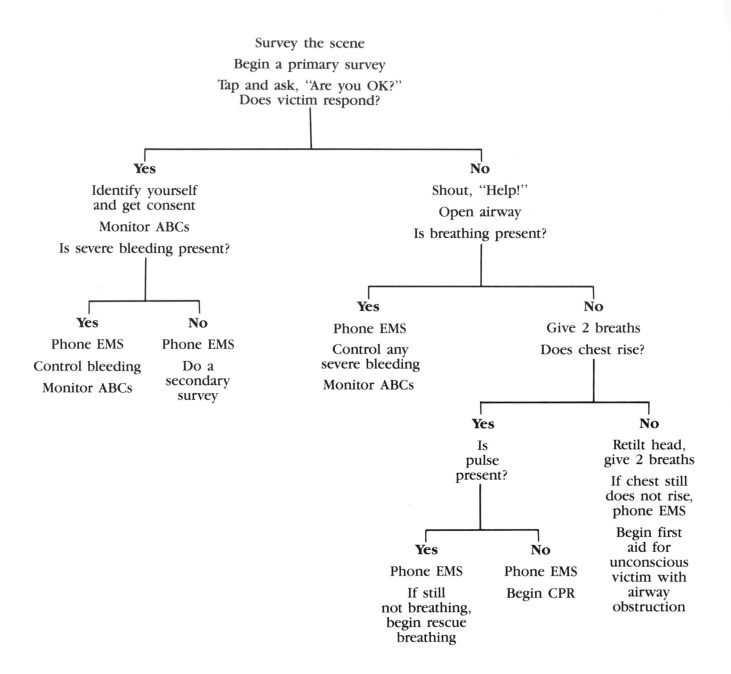

Survey the scene
Begin a primary survey
Tap and ask, "Are you OK?"
Does victim respond?

Yes

Identify yourself
and get consent

Monitor ABCs

Is severe bleeding present?

Yes

Phone EMS

Control bleeding

Monitor ABCs

No

Phone EMS

Do a
secondary
survey

No

Shout, "Help!"

Open airway

Is breathing present?

Yes

Phone EMS

Control any
severe bleeding

Monitor ABCs

No

Give 2 breaths

Does chest rise?

Yes

Is
pulse
present?

Yes

Phone EMS

If still
not breathing,
begin rescue
breathing

No

Phone EMS

Begin CPR

No

Retilt head,
give 2 breaths

If chest still
does not rise,
phone EMS

Begin first
aid for
unconscious
victim with
airway
obstruction

3 Choking (Airway Obstruction)

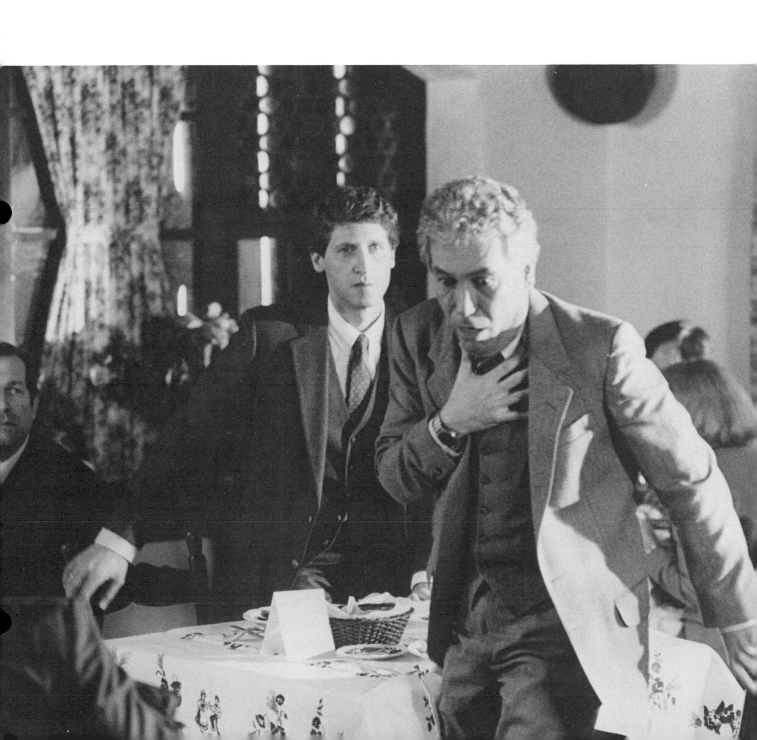

Choking (Airway Obstruction)

Learning Objectives

In this unit you will learn how to—
1. *Recognize when a person has an airway obstruction.*
2. *Perform first aid for a conscious victim with an airway obstruction.*
3. *Perform first aid for an unconscious victim with an airway obstruction.*

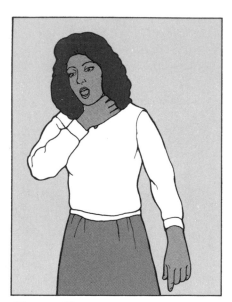

Figure 11
Universal Distress Signal for Choking

Definition

Choking, also known as airway obstruction, occurs when the airway becomes blocked due to a solid object, fluids, or the back of the tongue. A person who is choking may quickly stop breathing and lose consciousness.

Common Causes

About 3,000 people will choke to death this year. The most common causes of choking are—
- Trying to swallow large pieces of food that are poorly chewed.
- Drinking alcohol before or during eating. (Alcohol dulls the nerves that help you swallow.)
- Wearing dentures. Dentures make it difficult to sense the size of food when chewing and swallowing.
- Talking excitedly or laughing while eating, or eating too fast.
- Walking, playing, or running with objects in the mouth.

Signals

Being able to recognize when someone is choking is key to saving the victim. There are two types of obstructions that you need to know about—**partial airway obstruction** and **complete airway obstruction.** It is important to be able to recognize the differences between them.

1. Partial Airway Obstruction

   When a person has a partial airway obstruction, he or she can cough forcefully in an attempt to dislodge the object, and may be able to speak. He or she may also wheeze between breaths. The person may clutch at his or her throat with one or both hands. This is universally recognized as a **distress signal for choking (Fig. 11).** If the person is able to cough forcefully or is wheezing, do not interfere with his or her attempts to cough up the object. You should stay with the person and encourage him or her to continue coughing. If coughing persists, call EMS for help.

2. Complete Airway Obstruction

   A partial airway obstruction can quickly become a complete airway obstruction. A person with a completely blocked airway is unable to speak, breathe, or cough. Sometimes the victim may cough weakly and ineffectively or make high-pitched noises. All of these signals tell you the victim is not getting enough air to sustain life. Act immediately! Have a bystander call EMS personnel while you begin to provide care.

First Aid

Conscious Victim

To find out if a conscious person is choking, ask, "Are you choking?" If he or she is choking, then perform **abdominal thrusts** until the obstruction is cleared or the victim becomes unconscious. Refer to the skill sheets for Choking (Airway Obstruction)—Conscious Victim for the step-by-step procedure.

Unconscious Victim

To find out if the unconscious victim has an airway obstruction, begin with a primary survey to check the ABCs as you did for rescue breathing.

1. Check for unresponsiveness.
2. If no response, shout, "Help!"
3. Position the victim.
4. Open the airway.
5. Check for breathlessness.
6. If no breath, give 2 full breaths.
7. If you are unable to breathe air into the victim, retilt the victim's head and give 2 full breaths again.
8. Have someone phone EMS for help.
9. Perform 6 to 10 abdominal thrusts.
10. Do finger sweep.
11. Give 2 full breaths.

Repeat the last three steps until the obstruction is cleared or help arrives.

Refer to the skill sheets for Choking (Airway Obstruction)—Unconscious Victim for the step-by-step procedure.

Commonly Asked Questions About Choking

1. Q. Should I call EMS if the victim is conscious and the obstruction comes out easily and quickly?
   A. Yes. The object may cause tissues to swell and further complications might arise later.

2. Q. What if the unconscious person is too large for me to straddle?
   A. The best position for correct delivery of abdominal thrusts is to straddle the victim's thighs. However, you can straddle one of the victim's thighs instead of both, or you can kneel close to one side—but the thrust will not be as effective.

Skill Sheets: Choking (Airway Obstruction)

Conscious Victim

When practicing abdominal thrusts on a partner, do not give actual abdominal thrusts.

Partner Check
Instructor Check

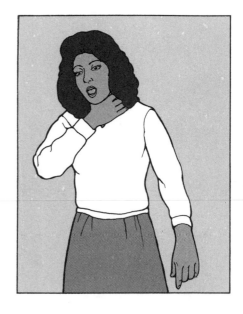

☐ ☐ **Determine if Victim Is Choking**

Ask, "Are you choking?"

If victim cannot cough, speak, or breathe, shout, "Help!"

Say, "I can help."

☐ ☐ **Phone EMS for Help**

Tell someone to call for an ambulance.

Say, "Airway is obstructed, call _____" (Local emergency number or Operator).

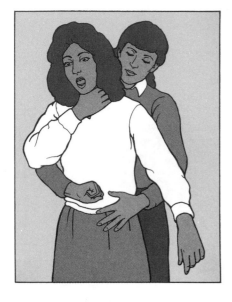

☐ ☐ **Perform Abdominal Thrusts**

Stand behind victim.

Wrap arms around victim's waist.

Make a fist with one hand and place thumb side of fist against middle of victim's abdomen just above navel and well below lower tip of **breastbone.**

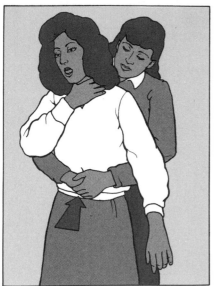

Grasp your fist with your other hand.

Keeping elbows out, press fist into victim's abdomen with a quick upward thrust.

Each thrust should be a separate and distinct attempt to dislodge the object.

Repeat thrusts until the airway obstruction is cleared or victim becomes unconscious.

Final Instructor Check _____

Skill Sheets: Choking (Airway Obstruction)

Unconscious Victim

You find a person lying on the ground, not moving. First, survey the scene to see if it is safe and to get some idea of what has happened. Then begin doing a primary survey by checking the ABCs.

Note: Before you practice on a manikin, clean its face and the inside of its mouth. The directions for doing this are found on page xii. Clean the manikin's face and mouth before each person in your group practices. Do not practice actual thrusts on your partner—only on a manikin.

Do not perform finger sweeps on a manikin. Do not touch the manikin's lips or inside of its mouth with your finger.

Partner Check
Instructor Check

☐ ☐ **Check for Unresponsiveness** (Does the victim respond?)

Tap or gently shake victim.

Shout, "Are you OK?"

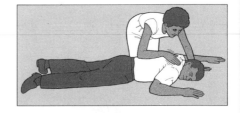

If no response, shout, "Help!"

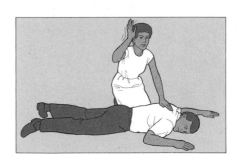

Choking (Airway Obstruction) Skill Sheets

Partner Check   Instructor Check

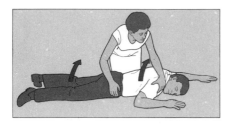

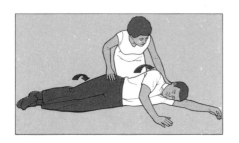

☐ ☐ **Position the Victim**

Roll victim onto back, if necessary.

Kneel facing victim, midway between victim's hips and shoulders. Straighten victim's legs, if necessary, and move arm closer to you above victim's head.

Place one hand on victim's shoulder and other hand on victim's hip.

Roll victim toward you as a unit; as you roll victim, move your hand from shoulder to support back of head and neck.

Place victim's arm nearer you alongside victim's body.

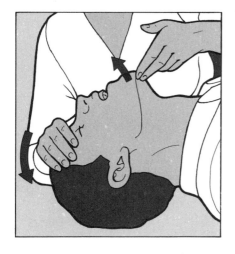

☐ ☐ **Open the Airway** (Use head-tilt/chin-lift method)

Place one hand on victim's forehead.

Place fingers of other hand under bony part of lower jaw near chin.

Tilt head and lift jaw. Avoid closing victim's mouth. Avoid pushing on soft parts under chin.

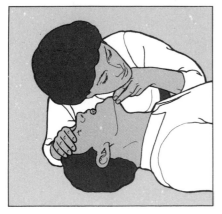

☐ ☐ **Check for Breathlessness** (Is victim breathing?)

Maintain open airway with head-tilt/chin-lift.

Place your ear over victim's mouth and nose.

Look at chest, listen, and feel for breathing for 3 to 5 seconds.

If no breath, say, "Not breathing."

34

☐ ☐ **Give 2 Full Breaths**

Maintain open airway with head-tilt/chin-lift.

Pinch nose shut.

Open your mouth wide, take a deep breath, and make a tight seal around outside of victim's mouth.

Give 2 full breaths. Each breath should last 1 to 1½ seconds. Pause between each breath for you to take a breath.

If you are unable to breathe air into the victim—

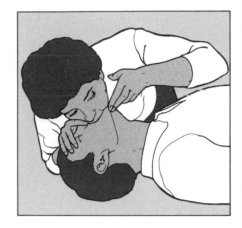

☐ ☐ **Retilt Victim's Head and Give 2 Full Breaths**

Retilt victim's head.

Pinch nose shut.

Open your mouth wide, take a deep breath, and make a tight seal around outside of victim's mouth.

Give 2 full breaths. Each breath should last 1 to 1½ seconds. Pause between each breath for you to take a breath.

If you are still unable to breathe air into victim—

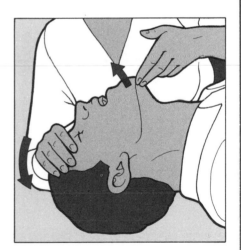

☐ ☐ **Phone EMS for Help**

Tell someone to call for an ambulance.

Say, "Airway is obstructed, call _____" (Local emergency number or Operator).

Choking (Airway Obstruction) Skill Sheets

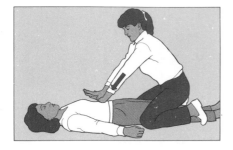

☐ ☐ **Perform 6 to 10 Abdominal Thrusts**

Straddle victim's thighs.

Place heel of one hand against middle of victim's abdomen just above navel and well below lower tip of breastbone.

Place other hand directly on top of first hand. (Fingers of both hands should be pointing toward victim's head.)

Press into victim's abdomen 6 to 10 times with quick upward thrusts. Each thrust should be a separate and distinct attempt to dislodge the object.

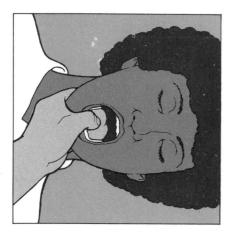

☐ ☐ **Do Finger Sweep (pretend)**

Move from straddle position and kneel beside victim's head.

With victim's face up, open the mouth and grasp both tongue and lower jaw between thumb and fingers of hand nearer victim's legs; lift jaw.

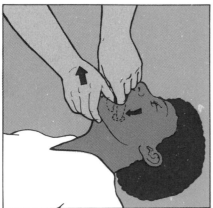

Insert index finger into mouth along inside of cheek and deep into throat to base of tongue.

Use "hooking" action to dislodge any object that might be there and move it into mouth for removal.

Say, "No object found."

Partner Check

Instructor Check

☐ ☐ **Give 2 Full Breaths**

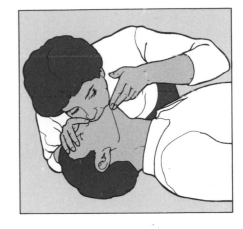

Open airway using head-tilt/chin-lift.

Pinch nose shut.

Open your mouth wide, take a deep breath, and make a tight seal around outside of victim's mouth.

Give 2 full breaths. Each breath should last 1 to 1½ seconds. Pause between each breath for you to take a breath.

If you are still unable to breathe air into victim—

☐ ☐ **Repeat Sequence Until Airway Is Cleared**

Do 6 to 10 abdominal thrusts.

Do finger sweep (pretend).

Give 2 breaths.

Final Instructor Check _____

Special Situations

Chest Thrusts

In some situations you may not be able to get your arms around the waist of a choking victim to deliver effective abdominal thrusts. For example, the person may be greatly overweight or pregnant. In the case of a woman in the late stages of pregnancy, abdominal thrusts could be dangerous. In both cases, **chest thrusts** are performed instead of abdominal thrusts. Chest thrusts are done in the following way:

- **Conscious Victim**

  With the person either standing or sitting—
  1. Stand behind the victim and place your arms under the armpits and around the chest.
  2. Place the thumb side of your fist on the middle of the breastbone *(Fig. 12)*.
  3. Grasp your fist with your other hand.
  4. Give thrusts against the chest until the obstruction is cleared or until the person loses consciousness *(Fig. 13)*.

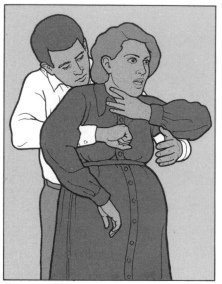

Figure 12
Hand Placement for Chest Thrusts

- **Unconscious Victim**

  Chest thrusts should be given only to an unconscious person who is in the late stages of pregnancy or who is greatly overweight. Follow the steps in the skill sheets for giving first aid for choking to an unconscious victim, but substitute chest thrusts for abdominal thrusts:
  1. Kneel facing the victim and place your hands as you would for CPR (pages 51–52).
  2. Give 6 to 10 thrusts. Each thrust should compress the chest 1½ to 2 inches. Give slow and distinct thrusts. Each thrust should be a separate and distinct attempt to dislodge the object.
  3. Do a finger sweep (page 36).
  4. Open the victim's airway and give 2 full breaths.

Repeat the last three steps until the obstruction is cleared or until EMS takes over.

When a Conscious Victim Becomes Unconscious

If a victim who is choking loses consciousness while you are giving abdominal or chest thrusts, you should shout for help and slowly lower the victim to the floor while supporting the victim from behind. Make sure the victim's head doesn't hit the floor.

Once you have lowered the victim to the floor, have someone phone EMS for help, if it hasn't already been done.
- Do a finger sweep.
- Open the airway and give 2 full breaths.
- Give 6 to 10 abdominal thrusts if you are unable to breathe air into the victim's lungs.

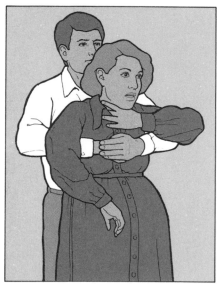

Figure 13
Giving Chest Thrusts

Repeat these three steps (finger sweep, rescue breaths, 6 to 10 abdominal thrusts) in the same sequence until the obstruction is cleared or until EMS takes over.

If You Are Alone and Choking

If you are choking and no one is around to help, you can do an abdominal thrust on yourself.

- Make a fist with one hand. Place the thumb side on the middle of your abdomen slightly above the navel and well below the tip of your breastbone.
- Grasp your fist with your other hand and give a quick upward thrust.

You can also lean forward and press your abdomen over any firm object that does not have a sharp edge—for example, the back of a chair, a railing, or a sink *(Fig. 14).*

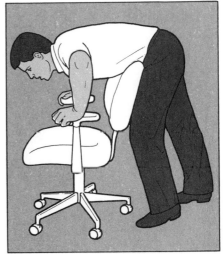

Figure 14
Self Abdominal Thrusts

Choking (Airway Obstruction) Action Guides

Conscious Victim

Survey the scene

Begin a primary survey

Ask, "Are you choking?"

Can the victim respond by coughing
forcefully, speaking, or breathing?

Yes

Identify yourself

If the victim is coughing forcefully,
encourage victim to continue coughing
and watch him or her until
obstruction is relieved

If coughing becomes weak
or ineffective, get consent

Phone EMS

Begin abdominal thrusts

Repeat until object comes out
or victim becomes unconscious

No

Shout, "Help!"

Say, "I can help you."

Phone EMS

Begin abdominal thrusts

Repeat until object comes out or
victim becomes unconscious

If victim becomes unconscious,
position victim on back

Begin first aid for an unconscious victim
with airway obstruction

Choking (Airway Obstruction) Action Guides

Unconscious Victim

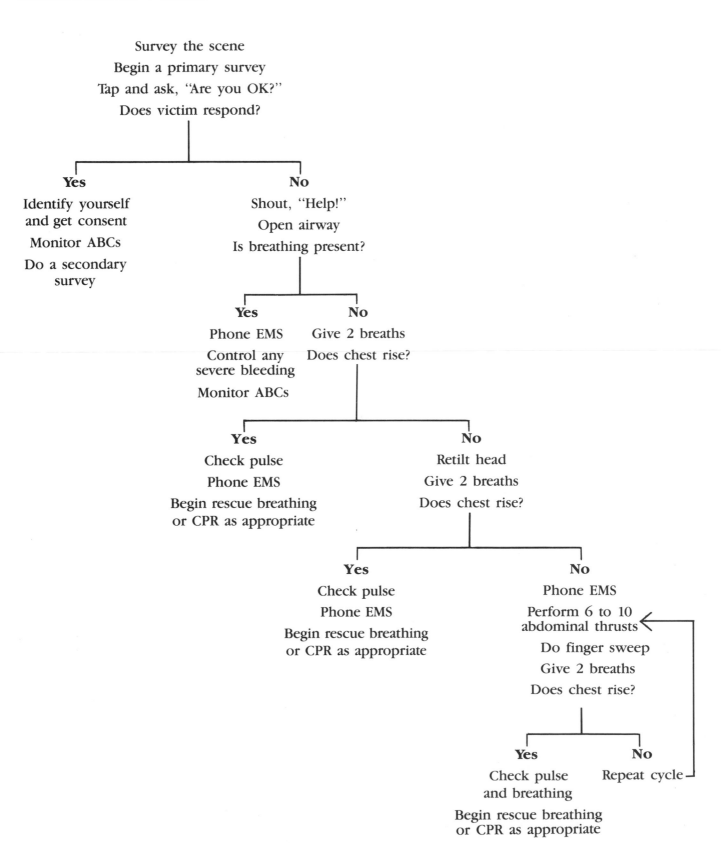

Survey the scene
Begin a primary survey
Tap and ask, "Are you OK?"
Does victim respond?

Yes

Identify yourself
and get consent

Monitor ABCs

Do a secondary
survey

No

Shout, "Help!"

Open airway

Is breathing present?

Yes

Phone EMS

Control any
severe bleeding

Monitor ABCs

No

Give 2 breaths

Does chest rise?

Yes

Check pulse

Phone EMS

Begin rescue breathing
or CPR as appropriate

No

Retilt head

Give 2 breaths

Does chest rise?

Yes

Check pulse

Phone EMS

Begin rescue breathing
or CPR as appropriate

No

Phone EMS

Perform 6 to 10
abdominal thrusts

Do finger sweep

Give 2 breaths

Does chest rise?

Yes

Check pulse
and breathing

Begin rescue breathing
or CPR as appropriate

No

Repeat cycle

4 Heart Attack, Cardiac Arrest, and CPR

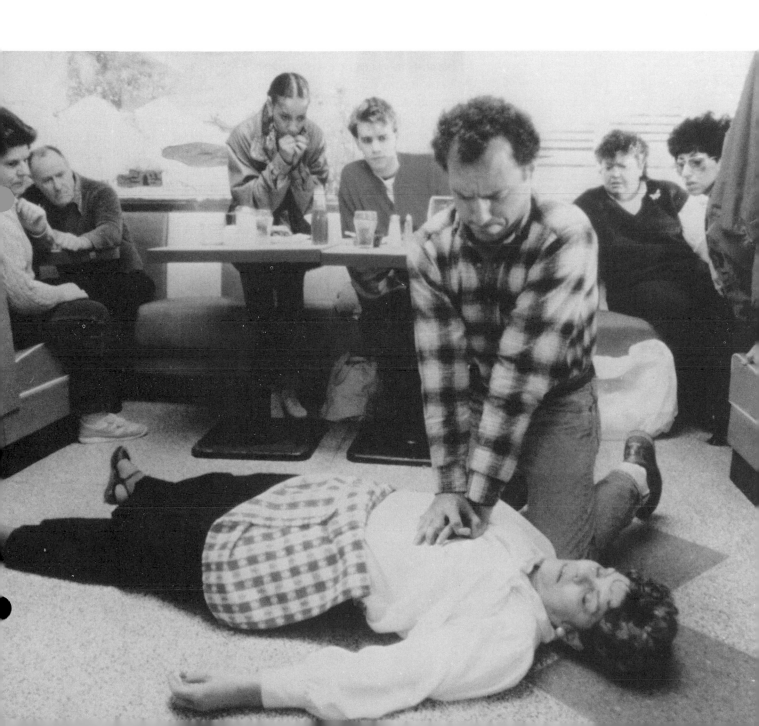

Heart Attack, Cardiac Arrest, and CPR

Learning Objectives

In this unit you will learn how to—
1. *Recognize the early warning signals of a heart attack.*
2. *Perform first aid for a heart attack.*
3. *Recognize a cardiac arrest emergency.*
4. *Perform CPR (cardiopulmonary resuscitation).*

Definition

A **heart attack** happens when one or more of the blood vessels that supply blood to a portion of the heart become blocked. When this happens, the blood cannot get through to feed that part of the heart and the cells begin to die. The heart may not be able to pump properly because part of it is dying.

If a large part of the heart is not getting blood, the heart may not be able to pump at all. If the heart stops, the victim is in **cardiac arrest;** and cardiopulmonary resuscitation (CPR—a combination of **chest compressions** and rescue breathing) must be started immediately.

Since any heart attack may lead to cardiac arrest, it is important to be able to recognize when someone is having a heart attack. Prompt action may prevent the victim's heart from stopping. A heart attack victim whose heart is still beating has a far better chance of living than someone whose heart has stopped. Most people who die from a heart attack die within 2 hours after having the heart attack. Many of these people could have been saved if the person having the heart attack, and the bystanders, had been able to recognize the signals of a heart attack and had taken prompt action.

Signals of a Heart Attack

The most significant signal of a heart attack is chest discomfort or pain. A victim may describe it as uncomfortable pressure, squeezing, a fullness or tightness, aching, crushing, constricting, oppressive, or heavy. The pain is described as being in the center of the chest behind the breastbone. The pain may spread to one or both shoulders or arms or to the neck, jaw, or back *(Fig. 15)*.

In addition to chest pain, other signals may include—
- Sweating.
- **Nausea.**
- Shortness of breath.

Many victims deny that they are having a heart attack. They may not want to admit to themselves or to others that they are having a heart attack. This denial may delay medical care when it is needed most.

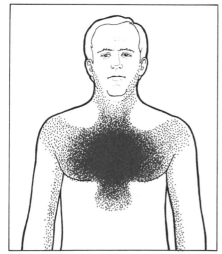

Figure 15
Areas for Heart Attack Pain

First Aid for a Heart Attack

A quick response in case of heart attack requires that you—
1. Recognize the signals of a heart attack and take action.
2. Have the victim stop what he or she is doing and sit or lie down in a comfortable position. Loosen restrictive clothing. Do not let the victim move around.
3. Have someone phone EMS for help. If you are alone, make the call yourself.

A key factor in whether or not a victim will survive a heart attack is how quickly the victim receives advanced care. Therefore, it is important to call EMS right away before the condition gets worse and the heart stops.

After EMS has been called, do a secondary survey. Ask the victim for information about his or her condition. Bystanders may also be able to give you some of this information. You should try to learn the following information:
- Victim's name
- Victim's age
- Previous medical problems ("Has anything like this ever happened to you before?")
- Where it hurts and how long the person has had pain
- Type of pain (for example, "dull," "heavy," "sharp")

Because the heart attack victim's heart may stop beating (cardiac arrest), you should be prepared to give CPR.

CPR—First Aid for Cardiac Arrest

If the heart does stop (cardiac arrest), the appropriate first aid begins with **cardiopulmonary resuscitation (CPR).** *Cardio* refers to the heart, and *pulmonary* refers to the lungs. So cardiopulmonary resuscitation means resuscitation of the heart and lungs. CPR is a combination of chest compressions and rescue breathing.

To help a person in cardiac arrest, you must provide CPR. CPR has two purposes. By breathing into the victim and compressing the chest, you—
- Keep the lungs supplied with oxygen when breathing has stopped.
- Keep blood circulating and carrying oxygen to the brain, heart, and other parts of the body.

How Heart Attacks Happen

While heart attacks seem to strike suddenly, the conditions that often cause them may build up silently for years. Most heart attacks are the result of cardiovascular disease. Cardiovascular disease happens when fatty substances and other materials build up in the blood and begin to stick to the walls of the blood vessels. Over time, the blood vessels get narrower. As the blood vessels get narrower, it becomes more and more likely that a blood vessel in the heart will become partly or completely clogged. This process can begin early in life; it may even begin in early childhood.

Cardiovascular disease may only be stopped or slowed by certain changes in the way you live. This disease cannot be stopped by medicines, though some related problems (like high blood pressure) can be controlled or slowed by medicines.

Risk Factors for Heart Disease

*Scientists have been able to identify certain things that are related to getting **cardiovascular disease.** They call these **risk factors;** some can be changed while others cannot.*

Risk Factors That You Cannot Change
- *Heredity (a history of cardio-vascular disease in your family)*
- *Sex (males are at a greater risk)*
- *Age (you are at greater risk as you get older)*

Heart Attack, Cardiac Arrest, and CPR

Risk Factors That You Can Change

- *Cigarette smoking*
- *High **blood pressure***
- *High blood **cholesterol** (influenced by a diet high in saturated fat and cholesterol)*
- *Uncontrolled **diabetes***
- *Obesity (being overweight)*
- *Lack of exercise*
- *Stress*

Unfortunately, there is no quick fix for dealing with the risk of cardiovascular disease. Just reading the list won't reduce your risk of having a heart attack. Reducing your risk requires effort on your part and guidance from your doctor or other health-care provider.

If you are interested in learning more about how to reduce your risk of cardiovascular disease, the American Red Cross can tell you about the resources available in your community to help you.

All of your body's living cells need a steady supply of oxygen to keep you alive. CPR must be started as soon as possible after the heart stops. Any delay in starting CPR reduces the chances that EMS personnel will be able to restart the heart. In addition, the brain cells begin to die after 4 to 6 minutes without oxygen.

The Technique

To find out if a person needs CPR, begin with a primary survey to check the ABCs as you did for rescue breathing. The skill sheets that follow provide the step-by-step procedure for giving CPR.

1. Check for unresponsiveness.
2. If no response, shout, "Help!"
3. Position the victim on his or her back on a firm, flat surface.
4. Open the airway.
5. Look, listen, and feel for breathing.
6. If the person is not breathing, give 2 full breaths.
7. Check the carotid pulse.
8. Have someone phone EMS for help.

If the victim is not breathing and has no pulse, give CPR. It is important that you check the victim's carotid pulse for 5 to 10 seconds before you start CPR because it is dangerous to do chest compressions if the victim's heart is beating.

To give CPR kneel beside the victim, lean over the chest, and find the correct position to give chest compressions. Give chest compressions by pressing down and letting up at a steady pace. Then give rescue breaths. These two steps keep oxygen-carrying blood flowing though the blood vessels.

Refer to the skill sheets for the step-by-step procedure for giving CPR.

Commonly Asked Questions About CPR

1. **Q.** Should I begin CPR if the victim has a very slow or very weak pulse?

   A. No. Performing chest compressions on a victim who has a pulse can result in serious medical complications. If no breathing is present but there is a pulse, perform rescue breathing and recheck the pulse frequently. If breathing and a pulse are present, maintain an open airway and keep checking both the breathing and pulse frequently.

2. Q. Does the victim's chest have to be bared to perform compressions? How much should be uncovered?

A. It is not necessary to bare the chest if the victim's clothing does not interfere with finding the proper location for chest compressions. If there are several layers of clothing, or if the clothing interferes with the performance of CPR, part of the chest should be bared. If possible, do not bare the entire chest, since a relatively small area is all that is needed for hand placement to give chest compressions. Most importantly, do not waste time or delay compressions.

3. Q. Can or should you do CPR on someone who has a pacemaker?

A. If a person's heart has stopped beating (no carotid pulse), CPR is needed to maintain blood circulation to the brain, heart, and other vital organs of the body. This is true regardless of whether or not the person has a pacemaker. Because the pacemaker is placed to the side of the heart and not directly below the breastbone, it will not get in the way of chest compressions.

4. Q. How long should I continue CPR?

A. Continue CPR until one of the following things happens:
- The heart starts beating again.
- A second rescuer trained in CPR takes over for you.
- EMS personnel arrive and take over.
- You are too exhausted to continue.

5. Q. Why is an electric shock used to restore the heartbeat when someone's heart has stopped beating?

A. In two-thirds of all cardiac arrests, the heartbeat flutters chaotically before it stops. The electrical impulses that cause the heart to pump fail to create the pumping needed to circulate the blood.

A defibrillator sends an electric shock through the chest to the heart to restore a functional heartbeat. Immediate CPR combined with early defibrillation give the victim of cardiac arrest the best chance for survival.

6. Q. What does "Phone First" mean?

A. The objective of the "Phone First" concept is to eliminate any delay in phoning for help in emergencies, especially cardiac arrest. Many people are slow to call EMS for help. They tend to confer with neighbors or family before deciding to call.

Someone who does not know what to do in an emergency should pick up the phone immediately and call for help. Calling the local emergency number will get medical help on the way, and the dispatcher will give instructions for care over the phone until help arrives.

Skill Sheets: CPR

Cardiac Arrest

You find a person lying on the ground, not moving. First, you should survey the scene to see if it is safe, and to get some idea of what has happened. Then do a primary survey by checking the ABCs.

Note: Before you practice on a manikin, clean its face and inside of its mouth. The directions for doing this are found on page xii. Clean the manikin's face and mouth before each person in your group practices. Do not practice actual compressions on your partner—only on a manikin.

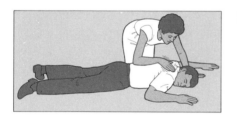

☐ ☐ **Check for Unresponsiveness** (Does the victim respond?)

Tap or gently shake victim.

Shout, "Are you OK?"

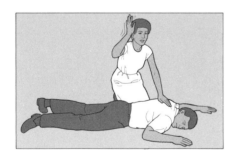

If no response, shout, "Help!"

☐ ☐ **Position the Victim**

Roll victim onto back, if necessary.

Kneel facing victim, midway between victim's hips and shoulders.

Straighten victim's legs, if necessary, and move victim's arm closer to you above victim's head.

Lean over victim and place one hand on victim's shoulder and other hand on victim's hip.

Roll victim toward you as a single unit; as you roll victim, move your hand from victim's shoulder to support back of the head and neck.

Place victim's arm nearer you alongside victim's body.

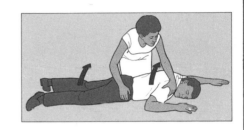

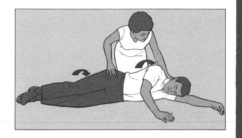

☐ ☐ **Open the Airway** (Use head-tilt/chin-lift)

Place one hand—the one nearer the victim's head—on victim's forehead.

Place 2 fingers of other hand under bony part of lower jaw near chin.

Tilt head and lift jaw. Avoid closing victim's mouth. Avoid pushing on soft parts under chin.

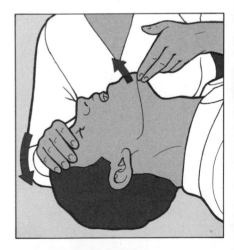

☐ ☐ **Check for Breathlessness** (Is breathing present?)

Maintain open airway with head-tilt/chin-lift.

Place your ear over victim's mouth and nose.

Look at chest, listen and feel for breathing for 3 to 5 seconds.

Say, "No breathing."

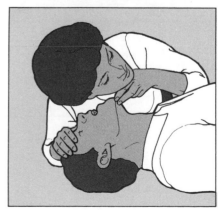

Partner Check
Instructor Check

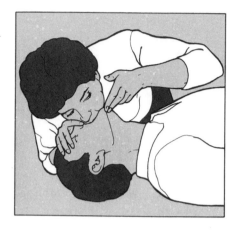

☐ ☐ **Give 2 Full Breaths**

Maintain open airway with head-tilt/chin-lift.

Pinch nose shut.

Open your mouth wide, take a deep breath, and make a tight seal around outside of victim's mouth.

Give 2 full breaths. Each breath should last 1 to 1½ seconds. Pause between each breath for you to take a breath.

Look for chest to rise and fall. Listen and feel for escaping air.

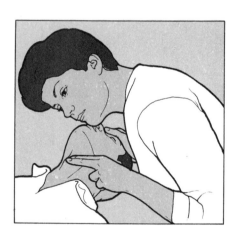

☐ ☐ **Check for Pulse and Severe Bleeding**

Maintain head-tilt with one hand on forehead.

Locate Adam's apple with middle and index fingers of hand closer to victim's feet.

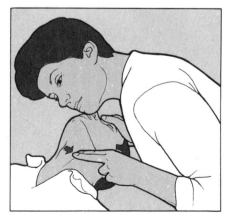

Slide fingers down into groove of neck on side closer to you.

Feel for carotid pulse for 5 to 10 seconds.

Look over victim's body quickly to see if he or she is bleeding severely.

Say, "No breathing and no pulse."

☐ ☐ **Phone EMS for Help**

Tell someone to call for an ambulance.

Say, "No breathing, no pulse, call _____ " (Local emergency number or Operator).

☐ ☐ **Locate Compression Position**

Kneel, facing victim's chest.

With middle and index fingers of hand nearer victim's legs, locate lower edge of victim's rib cage on side closer to you.

Slide fingers up edge of rib cage to **notch** at lower end of breastbone.

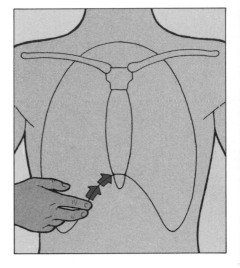

Place middle finger in notch, and index finger next to it on the lower end of breastbone.

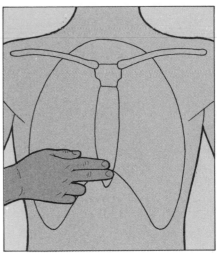

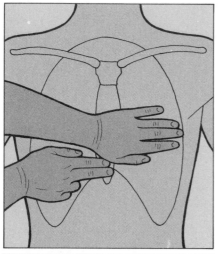

Place heel of hand nearer victim's head on breastbone next to index finger of hand used to find notch.

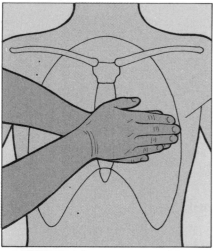

Place heel of hand used to locate notch directly on top of heel of other hand.

Keep fingers off victim's chest.

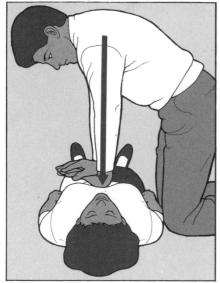

Position shoulders over hands, with elbows locked and arms straight.

Partner Check
Instructor Check

☐ ☐ **Give 15 Compressions**

Compress breastbone 1½ to 2 inches at a rate of 80 to 100 compressions per minute. (15 compressions should take 9 to 11 seconds.)

Count aloud, "One and two and three and four and five and six and . . . fifteen and." (Push down as you say the number and come up as you say *and*.)

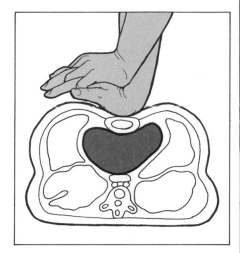

Compress down and up smoothly, keeping hand contact with chest at all times.

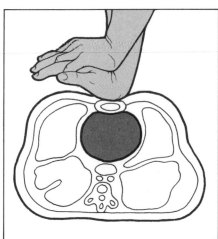

Partner Check

Instructor Check

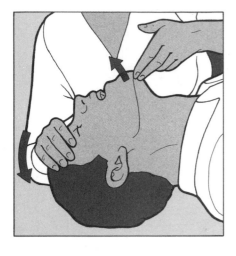

☐ ☐ **Give 2 Full Breaths**

Open airway with head-tilt/chin-lift.

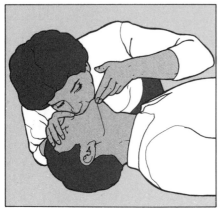

Pinch nose shut.

Open your mouth wide, take a deep breath, and make a tight seal around outside of victim's mouth.

Give 2 full breaths. Each breath should last 1 to 1½ seconds. Pause between each breath for you to take a breath.

Look for chest to rise and fall. Listen and feel for escaping air.

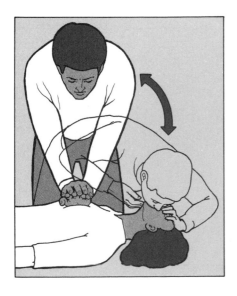

☐ ☐ **Do Compression/Breathing Cycles**

Do 3 more cycles of 15 compressions and 2 breaths.

☐ ☐ **Recheck Carotid Pulse**

Tilt head.

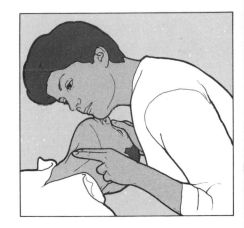

Locate carotid pulse and feel for 5 seconds.

Say, "No pulse."

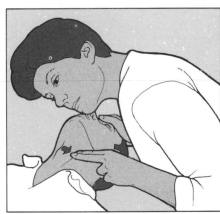

☐ ☐ **Give 2 Full Breaths**

Open airway with head-tilt/chin-lift.

Pinch nose shut.

Open your mouth wide and make a tight seal around outside of victim's mouth.

Give 2 full breaths. Each breath should last 1 to 1½ seconds. Pause between each breath for you to take a breath.

Look for chest to risc and fall. Listen and feel for escaping air.

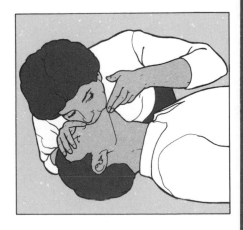

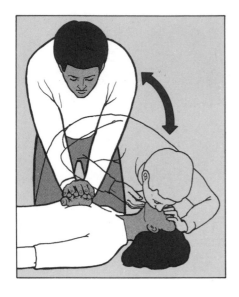

☐ ☐ **Continue Compression/Breathing Cycles**

Locate correct hand position.

Continue cycles of 15 compressions and 2 breaths.

Recheck pulse every few minutes.

☐ ☐ **What to Do Next**

If there is still no pulse, continue CPR.

If pulse returns, check breathing.

If victim is not breathing, begin rescue breathing.

If victim is breathing, monitor ABCs.

Final Instructor Check _____

Special Situations

If a Second Person Trained in CPR Is at the Scene

If another person trained in CPR is at the scene, this person should do two things: first, phone EMS for help if this has not been done; second, take over CPR when the first person is tired. Here are the steps for entry of the second trained person:

- Identify himself or herself as a person who knows CPR who is willing to help.
- If EMS has been called and if the first person is tired and asks for help, then:

  1. The first person should stop CPR after the next set of 2 breaths.
  2. The second person should kneel next to the victim opposite the first person, tilt the victim's head back, and feel for the carotid pulse for 5 seconds.
  3. If there is no pulse, the second person should give 2 breaths and continue CPR.
  4. The first person should then check the adequacy of the second person's breaths and chest compressions. This is done by watching the victim's chest rise and fall during rescue breathing and by feeling the carotid pulse for **artificial pulse** during chest compressions. This artificial pulse will tell you that blood is moving through the body.

Heart Attack, Cardiac Arrest, and CPR Action Guide

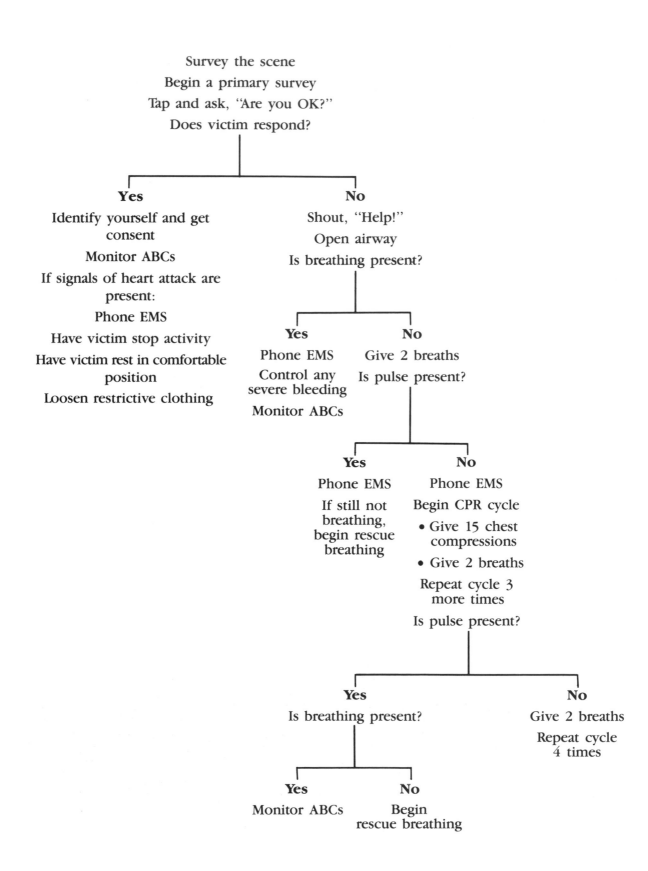

Survey the scene
Begin a primary survey
Tap and ask, "Are you OK?"
Does victim respond?

Yes

Identify yourself and get consent
Monitor ABCs
If signals of heart attack are present:
Phone EMS
Have victim stop activity
Have victim rest in comfortable position
Loosen restrictive clothing

No

Shout, "Help!"
Open airway
Is breathing present?

Yes

Phone EMS
Control any severe bleeding
Monitor ABCs

No

Give 2 breaths
Is pulse present?

Yes

Phone EMS
If still not breathing, begin rescue breathing

No

Phone EMS
Begin CPR cycle
• Give 15 chest compressions
• Give 2 breaths
Repeat cycle 3 more times
Is pulse present?

Yes

Is breathing present?

Yes

Monitor ABCs

No

Begin rescue breathing

No

Give 2 breaths
Repeat cycle 4 times

Section II

5 *Secondary Survey*

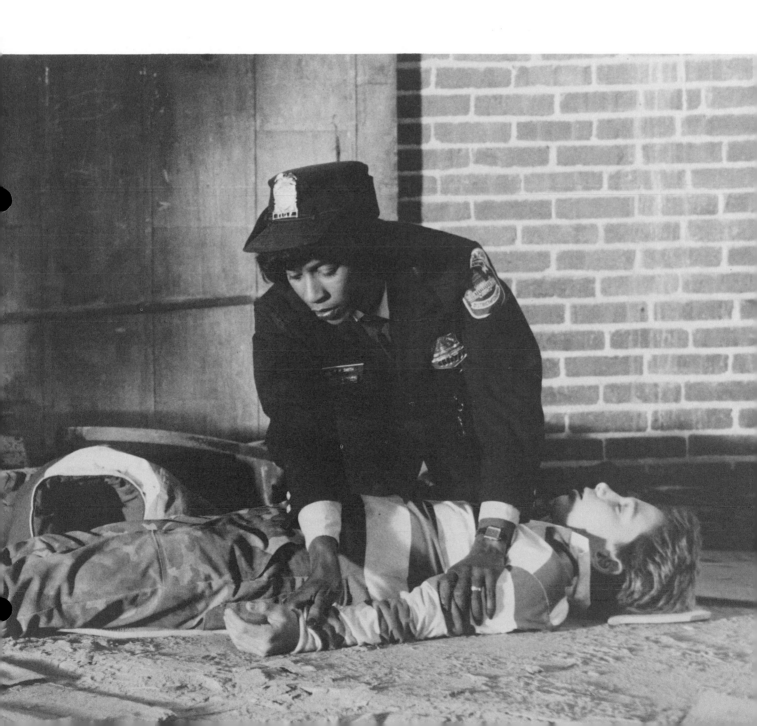

Secondary Survey

Learning Objective

In this unit you will learn how to do a secondary survey.

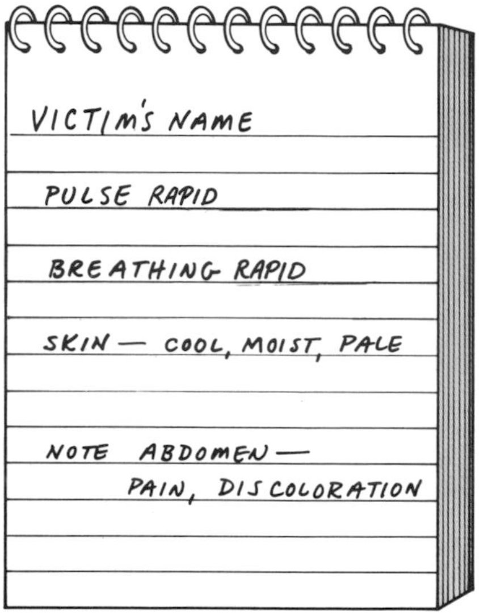

VICTIM'S NAME

PULSE RAPID

BREATHING RAPID

SKIN — COOL, MOIST, PALE

NOTE ABDOMEN —
      PAIN, DISCOLORATION

Figure 16
Writing Down Information

In Section I of this workbook, you covered the first three steps of the emergency action principles. You learned how to identify and care for life-threatening injuries a victim might have. In Section II, you will learn how to identify and care for further injuries a victim might have.

Section II begins with this unit on the secondary survey, the fourth step of the emergency action principles. The purpose of a secondary survey is to check the victim carefully and in an orderly way for problems that are not immediately life-threatening, but could become so if not cared for. As someone trained in basic first aid, you would do a complete secondary survey only on a fully conscious victim. If the victim is unconscious, you would stay at his or her head to monitor the ABCs until EMS arrives.

During a secondary survey, you look for important signals of possible injury or illness. A secondary survey has three steps.
1. Interview the victim and/or bystanders.
2. Check the victim's vital signs.
3. Do a head-to-toe exam.

If possible, you or a bystander should write down the information from a secondary survey *(Fig. 16)*. This will be helpful to EMS personnel later on.

When you do the secondary survey, remember not to move the victim. Most injured people will find the most comfortable position for themselves.

Victim and Bystander Interviews

This first step in a secondary survey gives you important information about what happened to the victim. It helps you determine what to look for while you complete the rest of the secondary survey.

Begin by identifying yourself as someone trained in first aid. Get the victim's consent to give first aid, and reassure him or her. Interview the victim first. Ask the victim his or her name and then use it. Build on what you learned in the survey of the scene. What else can you find out about the injury or illness? Ask the victim specific questions about how he or she feels. Ask if the victim has any pain or discomfort. Ask about any medical problems, allergies, and medications.

After interviewing the victim, ask bystanders what they saw and what they know about the victim.

If the victim is unconscious, stay at his or her head to monitor the ABCs. You can interview the bystanders from there.

The more you learn, the more you can help the victim and the more you can tell EMS about the illness or injury.

Vital Signs

A person's breathing, pulse, and skin characteristics are called vital signs. These vital signs can give you signals that tell you how the body is responding to injury or illness. Look for changes or any problems in breathing, pulse, or skin appearance and temperature. Note anything unusual. Check these vital signs about every five minutes until EMS personnel arrive.

Changes in Breathing

A healthy person breathes regularly. Breathing should be effortless and quiet. In the secondary survey, watch and listen for any changes in normal breathing. Abnormal breathing may indicate a potential problem. The signals of abnormal breathing include—

- Gasping for air.
- Noisy breathing, including whistling sounds, crowing, gurgling.
- Very fast or slow breathing. (Normal breathing for adults is 10 to 20 breaths per minute.)
- Painful breathing.

Changes in Pulse

When the heart is healthy, it beats with a steady rhythm. This creates a regular pulse. You can feel the pulse with your fingertips in arteries near the skin's surface. If the heartbeart changes, so does the pulse. An abnormal pulse may be a signal that indicates a potential problem. These signals include—

- Irregular pulse.
- Weak and hard-to-find pulse.
- Very fast or slow pulse. (Normal pulse for an adult is 60 to 100 beats per minute.)

A sick or injured person's pulse may be hard to find. If this happens, keep checking for a pulse periodically. Take your time. Remember, if a person is breathing, his or her heart is also beating. However, there may be a loss of pulse in the injured area. If you cannot find the pulse, check it in another major artery—in the other wrist or the neck.

Changes in Skin Appearance and Temperature

The appearance of the skin and its temperature often tell you something about the victim's condition. For example, someone with a breathing problem may have a flushed or a pale face.

1. Look at the victim's face. Is the skin red, pale, or bluish?
2. Determine the temperature of the skin by feeling it with your hand. Does it feel warm or cool? Does it feel moist?

Be especially alert for vital signs that indicate life-threatening conditions such as **shock** (see Unit 6).

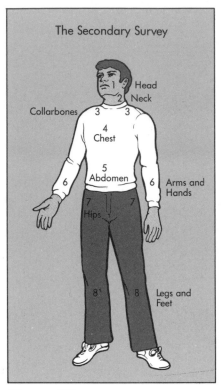

Figure 17
Order for Doing Head-to-Toe Exam

Head-to-Toe Exam

The last step of the secondary survey is the head-to-toe exam, which helps gather more information about the victim's condition. When you do the head-to-toe exam, use your senses—sight, sound, and smell—to detect anything abnormal. For example, you may smell an unusual odor that could indicate a victim has been poisoned or see a bruise or a deformed body part. Listen carefully to what the victim may tell you.

Begin by telling the victim what you are going to do. Ask the victim to remain still. He or she may move around but usually will not move a body part that is injured. Ask the victim to tell you if any areas hurt. **Avoid touching any painful areas or having the victim move any area in which there is discomfort.** Watch the victim's face, and listen for a tone of voice that may reveal pain. Look for a medical alert tag on a necklace or bracelet. It may tell you what might be wrong, who to call for help, and what care to give.

As you do the head-to-toe exam, think about how the body normally looks. Be alert for any sign of injuries. If you are uncertain whether your finding is unusual, check the other side of the body.

To do a head-to-toe exam, visually inspect the entire body, starting with the head *(Fig. 17)*. You might see abnormal skin color from bruising, a body fluid such as blood, or an unusual position of body parts. You may notice odd bumps or depressions. The victim may seem groggy or faint. Look for signs that may indicate a serious problem. If you see or suspect a condition that requires EMS personnel, call right away if you have not already done so.

Next, if you do not suspect an injury to the head or spine, determine if there are any specific injuries by asking the victim to try to move each body part in which there is no pain or discomfort. To check the neck, ask if the victim can slowly move his or her head from side to side. Check the shoulders by asking the victim to shrug them. Check the chest and abdomen by asking the person to try to take a deep breath and then blow the air out. Ask if he or she has any pain in the abdomen. Check each arm by first asking the victim if he or she can move the fingers and the hand. Next, ask if he or she can bend the arm. In the same way, check the hips and legs by first asking if he or she can move the toes, foot, and ankle. Then determine if he or she can bend the leg. Check only one arm or leg at a time.

If the victim can move all of the body parts without pain or discomfort and there are no other apparent signs of injury, have him or her attempt to rest for a few minutes in a sitting position. Continue to check the vital signs and monitor the ABCs. If no further difficulty develops, help the victim slowly stand when he or she is ready.

If the person is unable to move a body part or is experiencing pain with movement, or dizziness, recheck the ABCs. Help the person rest in the most comfortable position, maintain normal body temperature, and reassure him or her. Determine what additional care is needed and whether or not to call EMS personnel.

As you do this exam, keep watching the victim's level of consciousness, breathing, and skin color. If any problems develop, **stop** whatever you are doing, and give first aid **immediately.** The skill sheets at the end of this chapter give detailed steps for the secondary survey.

Provide Care

Once you complete the secondary survey, provide care for any specific injuries you find.

To provide care for the victim until EMS personnel arrive, follow these general steps—
1. Do no further harm.
2. Monitor the ABCs.
3. Help the victim rest in the most comfortable position.
4. Maintain normal body temperature.
5. Reassure the victim.
6. Provide any specific care needed.

Skill Sheets: Secondary Survey

You have already surveyed the scene, done a primary survey, and phoned the local emergency number. You are ready to begin a secondary survey of a conscious person.

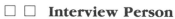

Partner Check

Instructor Check

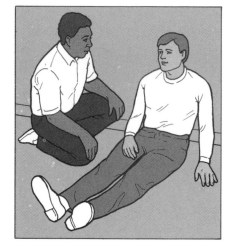

☐ ☐ **Interview Person**

Ask person. . .

His or her name.

What happened.

If he or she feels pain anywhere.

If he or she has any allergies.

If he or she has any medical conditions or is taking any medications.

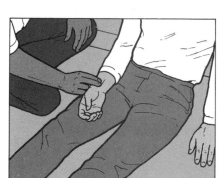

☐ ☐ **Check Vital Signs**

Determine if Pulse Is Abnormal

Tell person you are going to take his or her pulse.

Locate pulse on thumb side of wrist.

Ask yourself if it is—

Regular or irregular.

Hard to find.

Very fast or slow.

Note any abnormalities.

Partner Check
Instructor Check

Determine if Breathing Is Abnormal

Ask yourself if the person is—

Gasping for air.

Making unusual noises as he or she breathes.

Breathing very fast or slow.

Feeling pain when breathing.

Note any abnormalities.

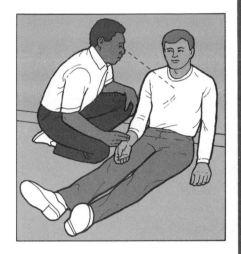

Determine Skin Appearance and Temperature

Feel person's forehead with back of your hand.

Look at person's face and lips.

Ask yourself if skin is—

Cold or hot.

Unusually wet or dry.

Pale, bluish, or flushed.

Note any abnormalities.

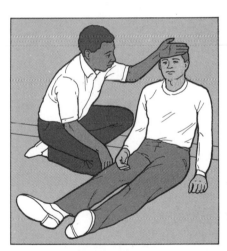

☐ ☐ **Perform Head-to-Toe Exam**

Note: Do not ask victim to move any area in which he or she has discomfort or pain or if you suspect injury to the head, neck, or back.

Visually Inspect Body

Look carefully for bleeding, cuts, bruises, and obvious deformities.

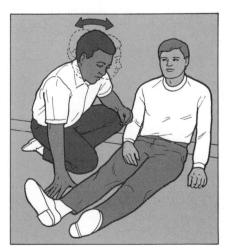

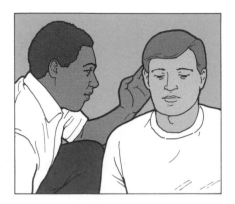

Check Ears, Nose, and Mouth

Look for fluid or blood.

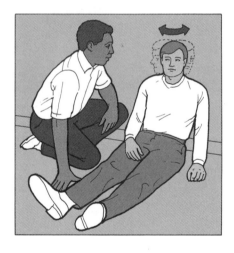

Check Neck

Ask person to move head slowly from side to side.

Note pain, discomfort, or inability to move.

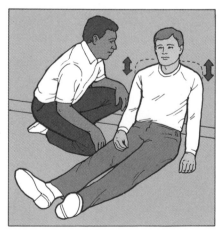

Check Shoulders

Ask person to try to shrug shoulders.

Note pain, discomfort, or inability to move.

Check Chest and Abdomen

Ask person to take a deep breath and blow air out.

Note any pain, discomfort, or inability to move.

Ask if person has pain in his or her abdomen.

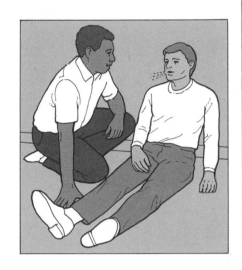

Check Arms

Check one arm at a time.

Ask person to try to—

    Move hands and fingers.

    Bend arm.

Note any pain, discomfort, or inability to move.

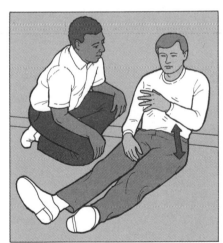

Check Hips and Legs

Check one leg at a time.

Ask person to try to—

    Move foot, toes, and ankle.

    Bend leg.

Note any pain, discomfort, or inability to move.

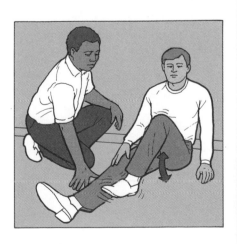

If person can move body parts without pain or discomfort or is not dizzy—

Have person sit up and rest for a few minutes.

If no further difficulty, have person stand slowly.

Determine if further care is needed.

If person is unable to move a body part or is experiencing pain on movement, or dizziness—

Recheck ABCs.

Help person rest in most comfortable position.

Maintain normal body temperature.

Reassure person.

Call EMS personnel for help if not already done.

Record Your Findings.

_____

_____

_____

_____

_____

Final Instructor Check _____

6 **Bleeding and Shock**

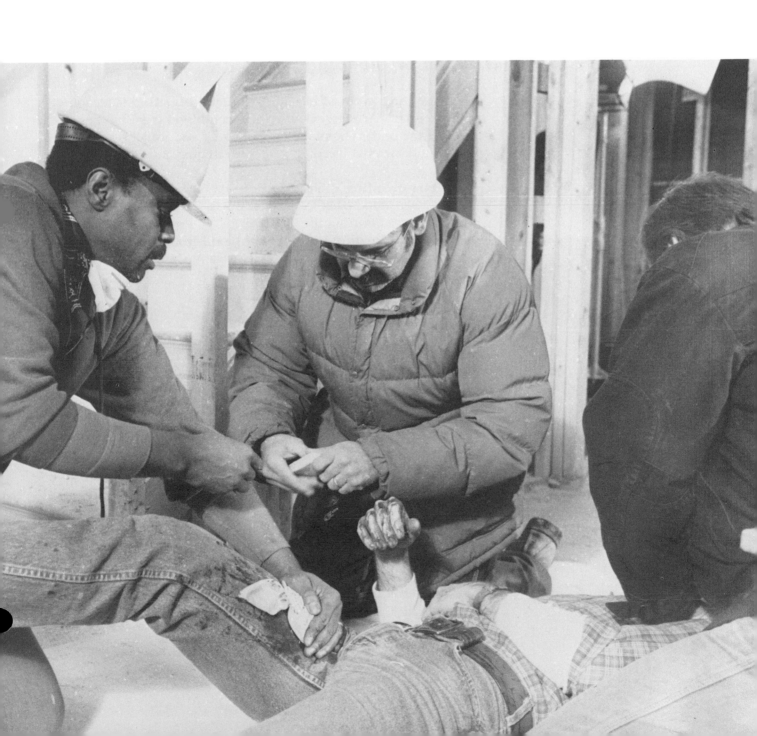

BLEEDING

Definition

Bleeding is the loss of blood from **arteries, veins, and capillaries.** Bleeding may be internal or external. Uncontrolled bleeding is life-threatening.

You check for severe bleeding during the primary survey, but you may not identify internal bleeding until you do the secondary survey.

Types of Bleeding

There are three types of bleeding. **Arterial bleeding** is bleeding from an artery. Arteries carry oxygen-rich blood from the heart through the body. The blood is bright red, and usually spurts from the wound. Arterial bleeding is life-threatening and is hard to control.

Venous bleeding is bleeding from the veins. Veins carry oxygen-poor blood back to the heart. It is dark red or maroon, and flows steadily from the wound.

Capillary bleeding is the loss of blood from capillaries, the smallest blood vessels. Blood flow is usually slow. It is often described as "oozing" from the wound.

External Bleeding

External bleeding occurs with open wounds. Open wounds are injuries that break the skin. The signals of life-threatening external bleeding include—
- Blood spurting from the wound.
- Bleeding that won't stop after all measures have been taken to control it.

There are four main types of open wounds: **abrasions, lacerations, punctures, and avulsions.**

Abrasions
An abrasion is the most common type of open wound. An abrasion occurs when the skin is rubbed or scraped away, for example, by falling on the hands or knees *(Fig. 18).* Abrasions are usually painful because sensitive nerve endings are exposed. There is usually little bleeding. However, because dirt and other matter can easily become embedded in the skin and cause infection, it is especially important to clean the wound.

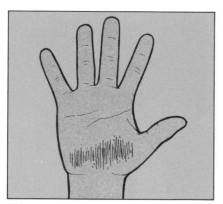

Figure 18
Abrasion

Lacerations

A laceration is a cut, usually from a sharp object. The cut may have either smooth or jagged edges *(Figs. 19 and 20)*. Lacerations are usually caused by sharp-edged objects such as knives or broken glass. A blunt force that splits the skin may also cause a laceration. Deep lacerations can damage nerves and blood vessels. Lacerations can bleed heavily. Because nerves may be damaged, lacerations are not always painful.

Punctures

A puncture wound results when the skin is pierced with a pointed object, such as a nail, a bullet, piece of glass, or a splinter *(Fig. 21)*. External bleeding is usually not severe, but there might be severe internal bleeding. There is a liklihood of infection with puncture wounds, particularly tetanus infection.

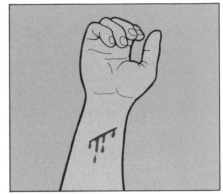

Figure 19
Laceration With Smooth Edges

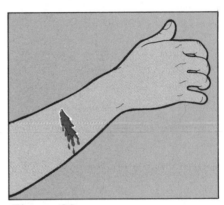

Figure 20
Laceration With Jagged Edges

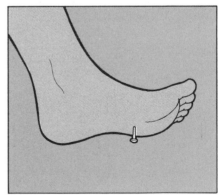

Figure 21
Puncture

73

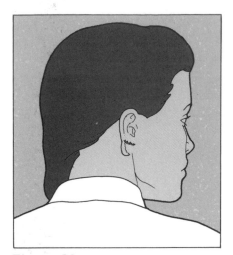

Figure 22
Partial Avulsion

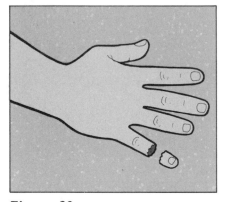

Figure 23
Complete Avulsion

Avulsions

An avulsion is an injury in which a portion of the skin and sometimes other soft tissue is partially or completely torn away *(Fig. 22).* Bleeding is usually significant.

Sometimes, a body part, such as a finger, may be torn completely from the body *(Fig. 23).* Although damage is severe, bleeding is usually not as bad as you might expect. Direct pressure will usually control it.

Avulsions may result from mishaps with machinery or explosions, for example. Often, the part can be reattached to the body. Wrap the part in sterile gauze, if any is available, or in a clean cloth. Place the wrapped part in a plastic bag. If possible, place the bag on ice to keep the part cool. Make sure the part is taken to the hospital with the victim.

First Aid for External Bleeding

To control external bleeding—

1. Place direct pressure on the wound with a dressing such as a sterile gauze pad or any clean cloth. Using a dressing will help keep the wound free from **germs.** Place a hand over the pad and press firmly. If a pad or cloth is not available, have the injured person apply pressure with his or her hand. As a last resort, use your own bare hand.
2. Elevate the injured part above the level of the heart if you do not suspect a broken bone.
3. Apply a pressure bandage to hold the gauze pad or cloth in place. Wrap the bandage snugly over the dressing to keep pressure on the wound.
4. If blood soaks through the bandage, add more pads. Do not remove any blood-soaked pads.

5. If bleeding continues, apply pressure at a pressure point *(Fig. 24)*. Make sure that EMS personnel are called.
6. Continue to monitor the ABCs. Watch the victim closely for signals that his or her condition is getting worse. Care for shock if necessary. If bleeding is not severe, provide additional care as needed.

The steps for bleeding control are illustrated in the skill sheets at the end of this unit.

Note that a tourniquet, a tight band placed around an arm or a leg to help constrict blood flow to a wound, is no longer used because it too often does more harm than good.

Preventing Disease Transmission

To reduce the risk of disease transmission when controlling bleeding, you should—
- Place an effective barrier between you and the victim's blood when you give first aid. Examples of such barriers are the victim's hand, a piece of plastic wrap, rubber or disposable gloves, or even a clean, folded cloth.
- Wash your hands thoroughly with soap and water immediately after providing care, even if you wore gloves or used another barrier. Use a utility or rest room sink, not one in a food preparation area.
- Avoid eating, drinking, and touching your mouth, nose, or eyes while providing care or before washing your hands.

Infection

Preventing Infection

When an injury breaks the skin, germs can get into the wound and cause infection. The first best way to prevent infection is to clean the area thoroughly. If the wound is not bleeding severely, wash the area with soap and water. Do not wash wounds that need medical attention because of tissue damage or heavy bleeding. They will be cleaned in the medical facility. It is more important for you to control bleeding.

Infected wounds can cause serious medical problems. Keep an up-to-date record of immunizations. The best way to prevent tetanus is to be immunized against it and to have a booster shot every 5 to 10 years or whenever a wound is contaminated by a dirty object such as a rusty nail.

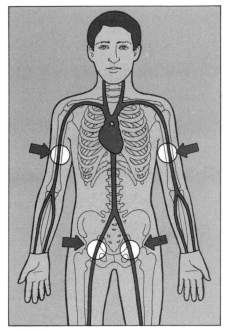

Figure 24
Location of Pressure Points

Signals of Infection

The early signals of infection are pain or tenderness at the wound, and redness, heat, or swelling. Some wounds may have a pus discharge. With more serious infections, red streaks may develop that lead from the wound toward the heart. The infection also may cause the person to develop a fever and feel ill.

Caring for Infection

If you see the early signals of infection, care for the wound by keeping the area clean, elevating it, and applying warm, wet compresses and an antibiotic ointment. Change coverings over the wound daily. If a fever or red streaks develop, the infection is worsening. If the infection persists or worsens, seek medical care without delay.

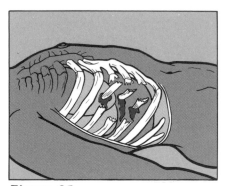

Figure 25
Internal Bleeding

Internal Bleeding

Internal bleeding is the escape of blood from arteries, veins, or capillaries into spaces inside the body, for example, into the abdomen. Internal bleeding ranges from small bruises beneath the skin to bleeding from deeper arteries and veins. Mild bruising is not serious, but bleeding from arteries and veins results in severe blood loss.

Severe internal bleeding usually occurs in injuries caused by a violent blunt force, such as in a car crash when the driver is thrown against the steering wheel. lt may also result from punctures or fractured bones. Both of these injuries can damage internal organs or blood vessels *(Fig. 25)*.

Signals of Internal Bleeding

Internal bleeding is harder to recognize than external bleeding. The signals are less easy to see and they may take time to appear. The signals of internal bleeding include—

- Bruising or discolored skin in the injured area.
- Soft tissues, such as those in the abdomen, that are tender, swollen, or hard.
- Anxiety or restlessness.
- Fast, weak pulse.
- Fast breathing.
- Skin that feels cool or moist or looks pale or bluish.
- Nausea and vomiting.
- Strong thirst.
- Decrease in level of consciousness.

First Aid for Internal Bleeding

1. If the injury seems to be a simple bruise, apply ice or a cold pack to help reduce pain and swelling. Always place a cloth between the ice or cold pack and the skin to prevent skin damage.
2. If you suspect more severe internal injury, the best help you can provide is to call EMS immediately. While you are waiting for help—
   - Do no further harm.
   - Monitor the ABCs.
   - Help the victim rest in the most comfortable position.
   - Maintain normal body temperature.
   - Reassure the victim.
   - Care for other injuries or conditions.

SHOCK

The body responds to injury or sudden illness in a number of ways. Shock occurs when the body cannot adjust to the stress placed on it by the illness or injury.

Definition

Shock is a condition in which the circulatory system (the heart, blood, and blood vessels) fails to provide adequate oxygen-rich blood to the body. When **vital organs,** such as the brain, heart, and lungs, do not receive oxygen-rich blood, they do not function properly. This results in shock. **Shock is life-threatening.**

Common Causes

Shock can be caused by sudden illness, such as a heart attack, or injury, especially injuries that result in severe bleeding. It can also result from emotional stress.

Signals of Shock

Shock victims usually show many of the same signals. These include restlessness or irritability; fast, weak pulse; fast breathing; pale or bluish, cool, moist skin; strong thirst; nausea and vomiting; drowsiness or loss of consciousness. If you recognize the signals of shock, give first aid immediately. **You do not have to identify what is wrong to give care that may help save the victim's life.**

First Aid

Follow the emergency action principles. First, check the ABCs. Care for any life-threatening conditions. Do a secondary survey if you do not find any life-threatening conditions. This is when you are most likely to identify the signals of shock.

Care for shock as follows:

- Do no further harm.
- Monitor the ABCs, and care for any airway, breathing, or circulation problems.
- Control any external bleeding as soon as possible.
- Elevate the legs about 12 inches if you do not suspect head or neck injuries, or broken hip or leg bones. Place the victim on his or her back and use available objects such as blankets, pieces of wood, boxes, and books to support the legs *(Fig. 26).*

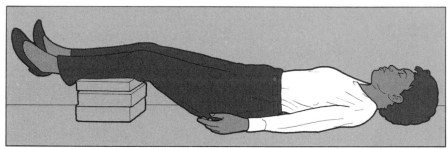

Figure 26
Usual Shock Position

- If you suspect head or neck injuries or if you are unsure of the victim's condition, keep him or her lying flat and wait for EMS *(Fig. 27).* Do not move the victim unless there is immediate danger from hazards such as fire, toxic fumes, heavy traffic, electrical wires, or deep or swiftly moving water. If you must move him or her, try not to bend or twist the body.

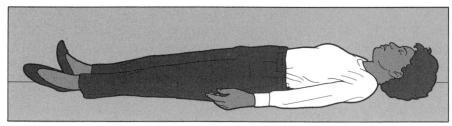

Figure 27
Shock Position: Suspected Head or Neck Injury

- If the victim vomits, place him or her on one side to avoid blocking the airway with any fluids *(Fig. 28)*. This position lets fluids drain from the mouth.

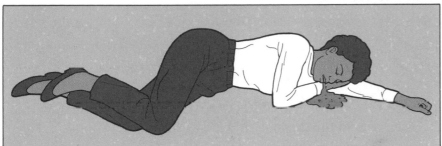

Figure 28
Shock Position: Victim Vomiting

- If the victim has trouble breathing, place him or her in a semireclining position, with boxes, pillows, or blankets raising the head and back *(Fig. 29)*. This makes breathing easier.

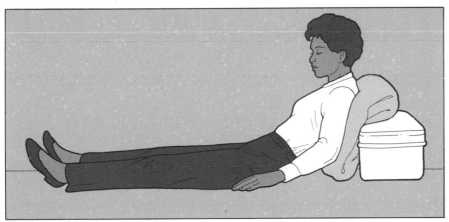

Figure 29
Shock Position: Difficult Breathing

- Help the victim maintain normal body temperature. Keep the victim from becoming chilled. Put blankets underneath and around the body, but do not overheat. If the victim is in a hot environment, try to cool him or her. For example, if the victim is outside on a hot day, provide shade and loosen clothing.
- Do not give the victim anything to eat or drink.
- Call EMS immediately. Shock needs professional medical care.

Skill Sheets:
How to Control External Bleeding

Forearm Wound

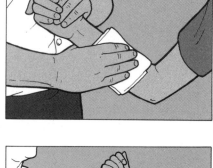

☐ ☐ **Apply Direct Pressure**

Place a sterile dressing or a clean cloth over wound.

Press firmly against wound with your hand.

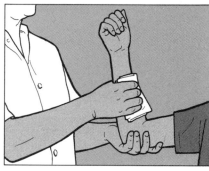

☐ ☐ **Elevate Body Part**

Raise wound above level of heart if you do not suspect a broken bone.

☐ ☐ **Apply a Pressure Bandage**

Using a roller bandage, cover dressing completely, using overlapping turns.

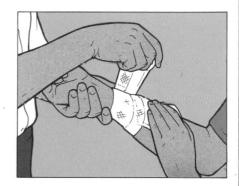

Tie or tape bandage in place.

If blood soaks through the bandage, place more dressings over the wound and bandage over them.

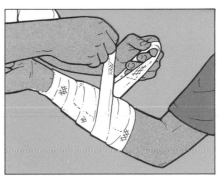

☐ ☐ **Apply Pressure to a Pressure Point if Bleeding Does Not Stop**

Maintain direct pressure and elevation.

Locate brachial artery.

Apply pressure to brachial artery by squeezing artery against underlying bone.

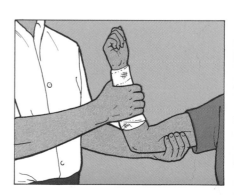

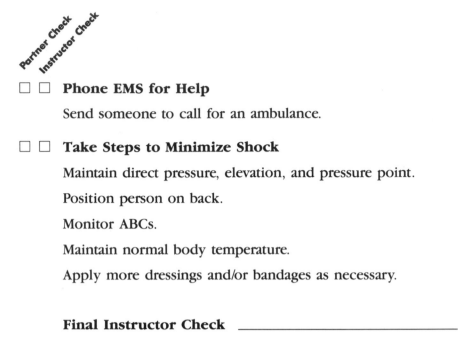

Partner Check   Instructor Check

☐ ☐ **Phone EMS for Help**

Send someone to call for an ambulance.

☐ ☐ **Take Steps to Minimize Shock**

Maintain direct pressure, elevation, and pressure point.

Position person on back.

Monitor ABCs.

Maintain normal body temperature.

Apply more dressings and/or bandages as necessary.

Final Instructor Check _____

Bleeding and Shock Action Guides

External Bleeding

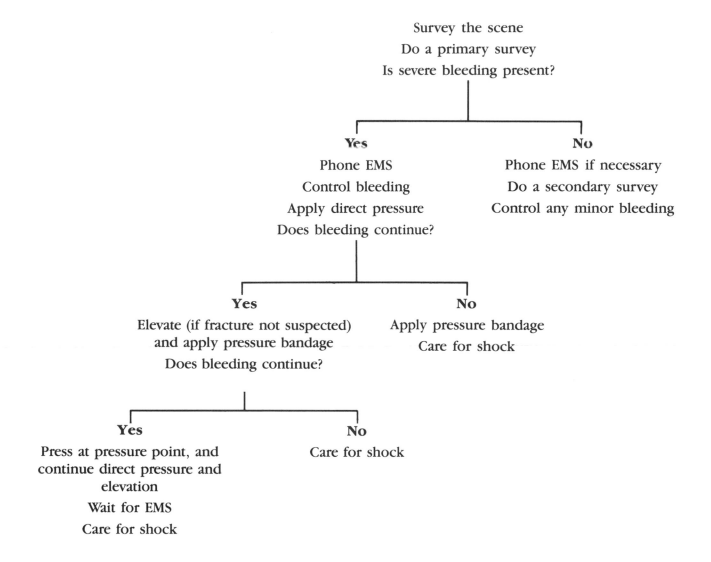

Survey the scene
Do a primary survey
Is severe bleeding present?

Yes
Phone EMS
Control bleeding
Apply direct pressure
Does bleeding continue?

No
Phone EMS if necessary
Do a secondary survey
Control any minor bleeding

Yes
Elevate (if fracture not suspected) and apply pressure bandage
Does bleeding continue?

No
Apply pressure bandage
Care for shock

Yes
Press at pressure point, and continue direct pressure and elevation
Wait for EMS
Care for shock

No
Care for shock

To reduce the risk of infectious disease transmission when you attempt to control bleeding, use some sort of barrier, such as several dressings, latex gloves, or a piece of plastic wrap. Always wash your hands as soon as you can after giving first aid. After touching one victim, always change the gloves or wash your hands before touching another to avoid cross-contamination.

Internal Bleeding

Survey the scene
Do a primary survey
Phone EMS
Do a secondary survey
Are signals of internal bleeding present?

Yes

Monitor ABCs

Reassure the victim

Control any external bleeding

Care for shock

If victim vomits,
place him or her on side

Care for other injuries or
conditions

No

Continue secondary survey

Signals of internal bleeding include bruising or discoloration in the injured area; tender, swollen or hard abdomen; anxiety or restlessness; fast pulse and breathing; cool, moist, pale, or bluish skin; nausea and vomiting; thirst; changes in consciousness.

Shock

Survey the scene

Do a primary survey

Phone EMS

Begin a secondary survey

Check vital signs

Are signals of shock present?

Yes

Care for shock:
- Position victim according to injury
- Maintain normal body temperature
- Control any external bleeding
- If victim vomits, place him or her on side
- Monitor ABCs

Are breathing and pulse still present?

Yes

Monitor ABCs

No

Begin rescue breathing or CPR, as appropriate

No

Complete the secondary survey

Care for any injuries or other conditions

Reassure victim until EMS arrives

Continue to monitor ABCs

Check for signals of shock

7 Burns

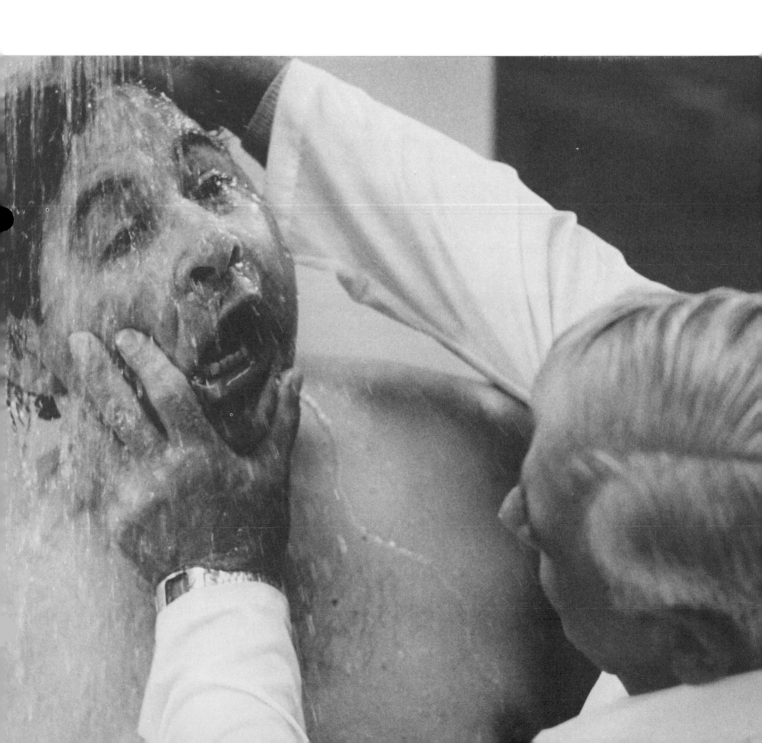

Learning Objectives

In this unit you will learn how to care for—
1. *Heat burns.*
2. *Electrical burns.*
3. *Chemical burns.*

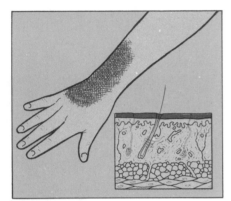

**Figure 30
First-Degree Burn**

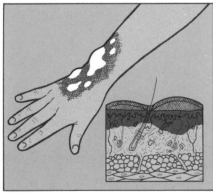

**Figure 31
Second-Degree Burn**

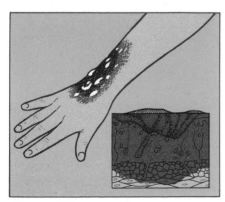

**Figure 32
Third-Degree Burn**

Definition

Burns are injuries resulting from exposure to heat, chemicals, electricity, or radiation. The severity of a burn depends on the temperature of the object or gas causing the burn, how long the skin was exposed to the source, the location and extent of the burn, and the victim's age and medical condition.

Common Causes

Burns have many causes, including carelessness with matches and cigarettes; scalds from hot water and other liquids; defective heating, cooking, and electrical equipment; unsafe use of flammable liquids to start fires and clean floors; unsafe use of strong alkalis such as lye, or strong acids; and fires. The hazards of fire include not only the visible burns but also respiratory and circulatory emergencies.

Types of Burns

Burns are classified according to their source, such as heat or chemicals, and their depth. The deeper the burn, the more severe it is. Generally, there are three depth classifications: first degree (superficial); second degree (partial thickness); and third degree (full thickness).

First-Degree Burns

First-degree burns involve only the top layer of skin *(Fig. 30)*. The skin is red and dry, and the burn is usually painful. The area may swell. Most sunburns are first-degree burns. First-degree burns usually heal in 5 to 6 days without permanent scarring.

Second-Degree Burns

Second-degree burns are deeper than first-degree burns. The burned skin will look red and have blisters *(Fig. 31)*. The skin may appear wet if the blisters are open. The burned skin may look mottled. Second-degree burns are usually painful, and the area often swells. The burn usually heals in three or four weeks. Scarring may occur.

Third-Degree Burns

Third-degree burns extend through the skin and into the structures below the skin *(Fig. 32)*. These burns may look brown or charred (black). The tissues underneath may look white. Third-degree burns can be very painful or may be relatively painless if the burn destroyed the nerve endings in the skin. The scarring that occurs may be severe. Third-degree burns are life-threatening.

Identifying Critical Burns

A critical burn is one which requires the attention of medical professionals. Critical burns are potentially life-threatening, disfiguring, or disabling. It is often hard to decide if you should call EMS for a burn injury. Call EMS for assistance immediately for the following burns:

• Burns whose victims are having trouble breathing
• Burns that cover more than one body part
• Burns on the the head, neck, hands, feet, or genitals
• Any second- or third-degree burn to a child or elderly person
• Burns resulting from chemicals, explosions, or electricity

First Aid for Heat Burns

If the scene is safe, do a primary survey. Call EMS, if necessary. Look for burns on the face, especially around the nose or mouth. If you see burns on the face, continually monitor the victim's breathing. These burns may signal that the airway or lungs are burned.

If burns are present, follow these four basic care steps:

• Cool the burned area.
• Cover the burned area.
• Prevent infection.
• Care for shock.

Cool the burned area immediately with lots of cool water. Do not use ice or ice water except on small first-degree burns. Apply wet cloths to an area that cannot be immersed.

Allow time for the burned area to cool. Continue cooling if the pain continues or if the edges of the burn feel warm to the touch when the area is taken out of the water. When the burn is cool, cut or carefully pull clothing away from the area. Do not try to remove clothing that is sticking to the skin.

Cover the burned area with dry, sterile dressings, if possible. Loosely bandage them in place. The bandage should not put pressure on the burn surface. If the burn covers a large area of the body, cover it with clean, dry sheets or other cloth.

Do not put ointments on any burn that will receive medical attention. Do not try to clean a third-degree burn. To prevent infection, do not break blisters.

Third-degree burns can cause shock as a result of pain and loss of body fluids. To minimize shock, lay the victim down unless he or she is having trouble breathing. Elevate the burned area above the level of the heart, if possible. Help the victim maintain normal body temperature.

Care for small first-degree burns and burns with open blisters that are not severe enough to require medical attention as follows:
• Wash the area with soap and water and keep the area clean.
• Apply an antibiotic ointment.
• Watch for signals of infection.

First Aid for Chemical Burns

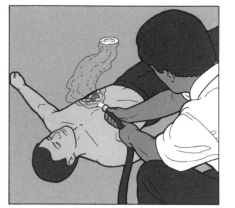

Figure 33
Flushing a Chemical Burn

If the scene is safe, do a primary survey. Call EMS. Use lots of cool, running water to flush chemicals from the skin *(Fig. 33).* Keep flushing with water until EMS personnel arrive. Remove clothing or jewelry on which chemicals have spilled, if possible. Care for possible shock, and monitor the ABCs.

If an eye is burned by a chemical, flush the eye with water until EMS personnel arrive.

First Aid for Electrical Burns

The signals of electrical injury include—
• Unconsciousness.
• Dazed, confused behavior.
• Obvious burns on the skin surface.
• Trouble breathing.
• Weak, irregular, or absent pulse.
• Burns both where the current entered and where it exited, often on the hand or foot.

Never approach a victim of an electrical injury until you are sure the power is turned off. If there is a downed power line, **wait for the fire department and the power company.** Do not touch downed power lines. If the emergency is inside, turn off the electricity at the fuse box or circuit breaker. This means you and others should know where the fuse box or circuit breakers are. Keep bystanders well away from any source of live current.

To care for a victim of an electrical injury, make sure the scene is safe. Call EMS immediately. Do a primary survey. Be aware that the victim may have trouble breathing or may be in cardiac arrest. As you do the secondary survey, check for more than one burn site. Cover all burns with dry, sterile dressings and care for shock.

A victim of lightning may have a life-threatening condition. He or she may not be breathing or may be in cardiac arrest. The victim may also have fractures, including a fractured spine, so do not move him or her. Any burns are a lesser problem.

Radiation Burns

Both the solar radiation of the sun and other types of radiation can cause burns. Sunburns are similar to heat burns. Usually they are mild but they can be painful. They may blister. Care for sunburns as you would for any other burn. Cool the burn and protect the burned area by staying out of the sun.

People are rarely exposed to other types of radiation unless they work in special settings such as certain medical, industrial, or research settings. People who work in such settings are provided training to teach them how to prevent and respond to such emergencies. If, however, you believe there has been exposure to radiation, contact EMS or civil defense authorities in your community *(Fig. 34)*.

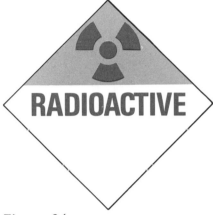

Figure 34
Radiation Emblem

Commonly Asked Questions About Burns

1. **Q.** Is it a good idea to put butter or oil on a burn?
    A. No. It would have to be removed before any medical treatment could be performed. Also, butter can contaminate the burn site.

2. **Q.** What about brushing dry chemicals such as lime off the skin?
    A. Do not brush dry chemicals off the skin unless large amounts of water are not available. It is possible that some chemicals might get into the eyes and burn them while you are brushing the chemicals off. On the other hand, some chemicals like lime become activated when only a little water is added. Because of these dangers, observe the following precautions when caring for burns caused by dry chemicals such as lime:
    * Rinse with large amounts of running water until EMS arrives.
    * If large amounts of water are not available, brush chemicals off skin.
    * If chemicals are near the eyes (on the face, neck, or shoulders) and large amounts of water are not available, have the victim close his or her eyes before you brush off the chemicals.

3. **Q.** As a person trained in first aid, should you try to neutralize a chemical burn?
    A. No. Combining acid and alkaline chemicals creates heat and could make injuries worse. Also, you don't have time to find a neutralizing agent. Use water.

Heat Burns

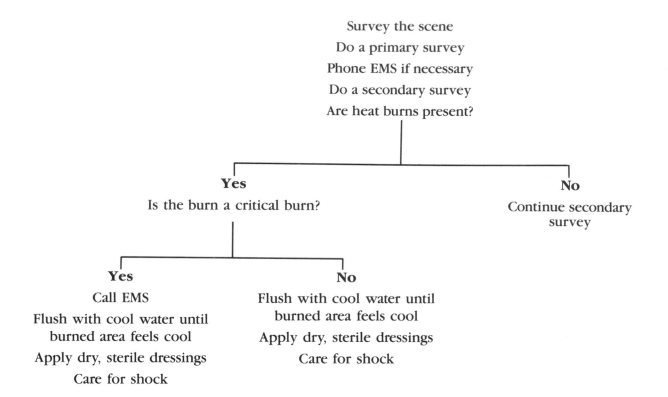

Survey the scene
Do a primary survey
Phone EMS if necessary
Do a secondary survey
Are heat burns present?

Yes
Is the burn a critical burn?

No
Continue secondary
survey

Yes
Call EMS
Flush with cool water until
burned area feels cool
Apply dry, sterile dressings
Care for shock

No
Flush with cool water until
burned area feels cool
Apply dry, sterile dressings
Care for shock

For a nonsevere burn, wash, apply an antibiotic
ointment, and watch for signals of infection.
If you suspect the victim has inhaled smoke
or chemicals (victim is hoarse and wheezing, breath
smells like smoke), remove victim from source
of injury if it is safe for you to do so,
monitor ABCs, and phone EMS.

Chemical Burns

Survey the scene

Do a primary survey

Phone EMS

Do a secondary survey

Are chemical burns present?

Yes

Flush immediately with large amounts of water. Continue flushing until EMS arrives

Remove any affected clothing or jewelry

Care for shock

No

Continue secondary survey

Electrical Burns

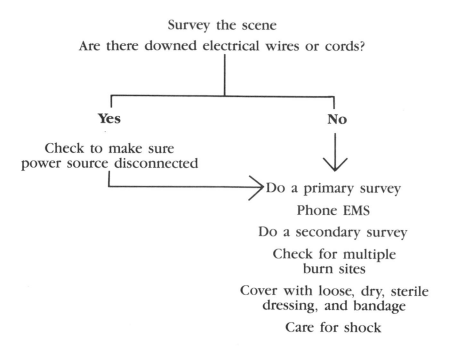

Survey the scene
Are there downed electrical wires or cords?

Yes   **No**

Check to make sure
power source disconnected

→Do a primary survey

Phone EMS

Do a secondary survey

Check for multiple
burn sites

Cover with loose, dry, sterile
dressing, and bandage

Care for shock

In electrical emergencies, check for the source of
electrical current. If inside, turn off the current at the
fuse box or circuit breaker. If outside, call the power
company. Never touch downed power lines. Keep
bystanders well away from live current.

8 Eye and Nose Injuries

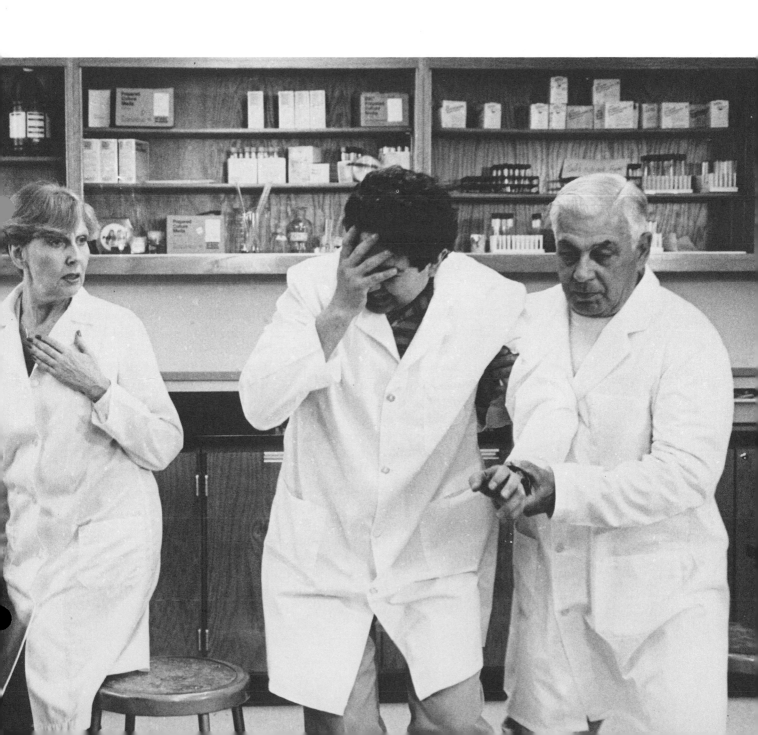

Eye and Nose Injuries

Learning Objectives

In this unit you will learn how to—
1. *Care for a chemical burn in an eye.*
2. *Care for a cut or an object in an eye.*
3. *Control a nosebleed.*
4. *Care for an object in the nose.*

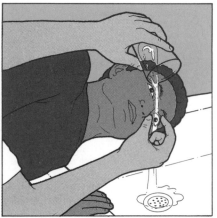

Figure 35
Care for Eye: Chemical Burn

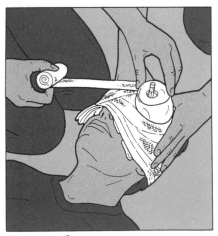

Figure 36
Care for Eye: Embedded Object

EYE INJURIES

Injuries to the eye can involve the bone and the tissue surrounding the eye, or the eyeball.

Common Causes

Blunt objects like a fist may injure the eye area, or a smaller object may penetrate the eyeball. Foreign bodies that get in the eye, such as dirt, sand, or slivers of wood or metal, are irritating and can cause a lot of damage.

Signals

The eye produces tears immediately in an attempt to flush out foreign objects. The irritation may be very painful. The victim may have difficulty opening the eye because light irritates it more.

First Aid

First, try to remove the foreign body by telling the victim to blink several times. Then try gently flushing the eye with water. If the object remains, the victim should receive professional medical attention.

Flushing the eye with water is also appropriate if the victim has any chemical in his or her eye *(Fig. 35)*. The eye should be continuously flushed until EMS personnel arrive.

Care for open or closed wounds **around** the eyeball as you would for any other soft tissue injury (see Unit 6).

Injury to the eyeball itself requires different care. Injuries that penetrate the eyeball or cause the eye to be removed from its socket are very serious and can cause blindness. Call EMS immediately. Never put direct pressure on the eyeball. Instead, provide care as follows:
1. Place the victim on his or her back.
2. Do not attempt to remove any object that has entered the eyeball.
3. Place a sterile dressing around the object.
4. Stabilize any impaled object in place as best you can. You can do this by using a paper cup to support the object *(Fig. 36)*.
5. Close and cover the unaffected eye to keep blood, fluid, or dirt from entering.

NOSE INJURIES

Severe nosebleeds can be frightening to the victim. It is possible that enough blood can be lost to cause shock.

Common Causes

Nose injuries are usually caused by a blow from a blunt object. The result is often a nosebleed. High blood pressure or changes in altitude can also cause nosebleeds.

First Aid

To control a nosebleed have the victim sit with the head slightly forward, chin toward chest. Then pinch the nose shut *(Fig. 37)*. Bleeding can also be controlled by applying an ice pack to the bridge of the nose or putting pressure on the upper lip just beneath the nose.

Once you have controlled the bleeding, tell the victim to avoid rubbing, blowing, or picking the nose, since this could restart the bleeding. Later, you may apply a little petroleum jelly inside the nostril to help keep it moist.

The victim should seek medical care if the nosebleed continues after you use the techniques described, if bleeding starts again, or if the victim says the bleeding is the result of high blood pressure. If the victim loses consciousness, place the victim on his or her side to allow blood to drain from the nose. Call EMS immediately.

If you think an object is in the nose, look into the nostril. If you see the object and can easily grasp it, then do so. However, do not probe the nostril with your finger. This may push the object farther into the nose and cause bleeding or make it more difficult to remove later. If the object cannot be removed easily, the victim should receive medical care.

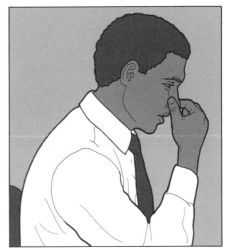

Figure 37
Controlling Nosebleed

A Commonly Asked Question About Nose Injuries

1. **Q.** Why shouldn't we stop a nosebleed by tilting the head back?
   A. If the head is tilted back, blood may collect in the stomach and nauseate the victim. This could cause vomiting, which would make first aid more difficult.

Eye Injuries

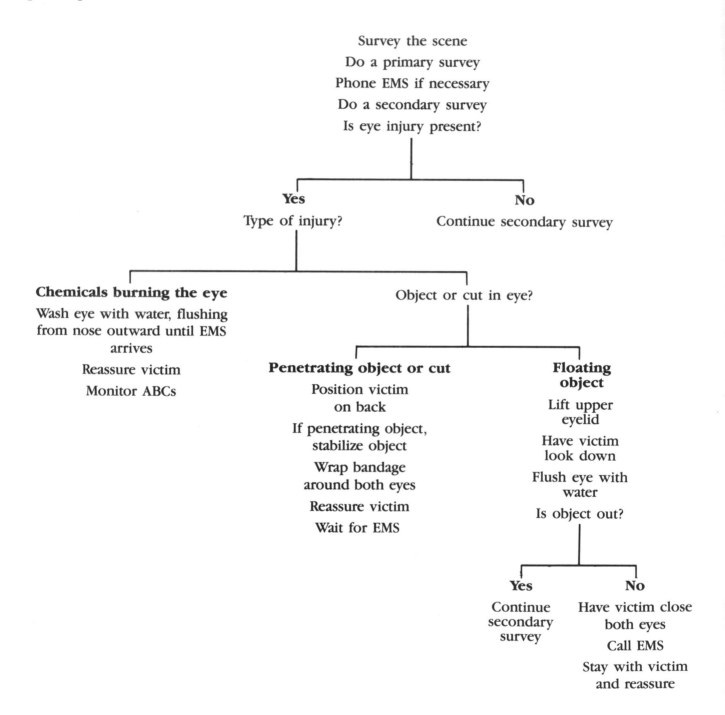

Survey the scene
Do a primary survey
Phone EMS if necessary
Do a secondary survey
Is eye injury present?

Yes
Type of injury?

No
Continue secondary survey

Chemicals burning the eye
Wash eye with water, flushing from nose outward until EMS arrives
Reassure victim
Monitor ABCs

Object or cut in eye?

Penetrating object or cut
Position victim on back
If penetrating object, stabilize object
Wrap bandage around both eyes
Reassure victim
Wait for EMS

Floating object
Lift upper eyelid
Have victim look down
Flush eye with water
Is object out?

Yes
Continue secondary survey

No
Have victim close both eyes
Call EMS
Stay with victim and reassure

98

Nose Injuries

Survey the scene
Do a primary survey
Phone EMS if necessary
Do a secondary survey
Is nosebleed present?

Yes

Have victim sit down

Lean victim forward with
chin toward chest

Pinch nose

No

Continue secondary survey

Nose injuries can indicate a possible head, neck, or back injury. Signals of such injuries can include any or all of these: pain and swelling, unequal pupil size, blood or clear fluid draining from the nose or ears, bruising under the eyes or behind the ears, loss of feeling in hands or feet, and an inability to move hands or feet. If you suspect a head, neck, or back injury, do not move the victim or stop the flow of blood and clear fluids coming from the nose or ears.

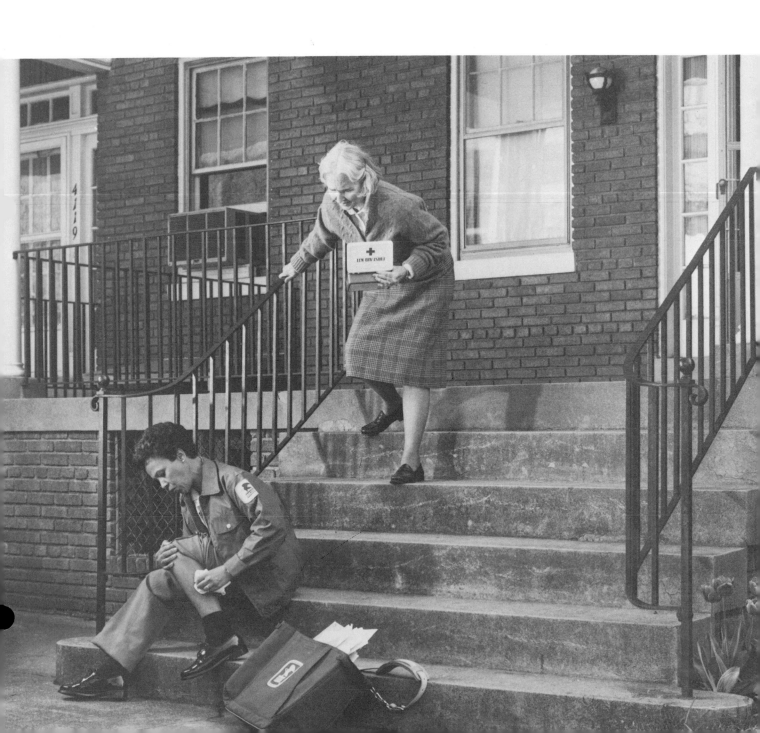

Learning Objectives

In this unit you will learn how to care for—
1. *Human and animal bites.*
2. *Insect bites and stings.*
3. *Allergic reactions to bites and stings.*
4. *Snakebites.*

HUMAN AND ANIMAL BITES

The mouths of people and animals are full of bacteria. A person who is bitten runs a high risk of infection. In general, people who are bitten by animals or other people should get medical help. They should also check to see if they have had a tetanus immunization within the last 5 years.

First Aid

If someone is bitten by an animal, try to get him or her away from the animal without putting yourself in danger. Do not try to restrain or capture it.

If the wound is not bleeding heavily, wash it with soap and water. Then control any bleeding and apply an antibiotic ointment and a dressing. Watch for signals of infection (described in Unit 6). The victim should get medical help if any of these signals develop.

If the wound is bleeding heavily, control the bleeding first. Leave the dressing and bandage in place. Do not clean the wound. The victim should get medical help. The wound will be cleaned by medical personnel. Remember to follow the guidelines for preventing disease transmission on pages x-xi when you are giving first aid.

Rabies

Rabies is an extremely serious illness transmitted to people through the saliva of diseased animals such as skunks, bats, raccoons, cattle, cats, dogs, and foxes. This can happen when a diseased animal bites people or licks open wounds on them. Since there is no proven cure for rabies, a person who is bitten by an animal that may be rabid must get medical help. If the animal is rabid, a series of shots (vaccines) must be given to the victim in order to build up body immunity in time to prevent the disease.

Animals with rabies act in unusual ways. For example, a wild animal with rabies might not run away from people. A rabid animal sometimes drools. Sometimes it acts irritable or strangely quiet. It might be partly paralyzed.

If you think an animal that has bitten someone is rabid, notify EMS, the police, and animal control. Tell the proper authorities what the animal looked like and where it was. They will capture it and then watch for signs of rabies. Never try to restrain the animal yourself. Keep away from it.

INSECT BITES AND STINGS

Insect bites and stings are very common. Although they can be painful, they rarely cause death. However, some people have a severe **allergic reaction** to an insect bite or sting that can result in a life-threatening condition. Signals of this allergic reaction and first aid are discussed later in this unit.

Tick Bites

Ticks can pass disease to humans. Much attention is now given to a new disease transmitted by ticks called Lyme disease. Lyme disease is an illness that people get from the bite of an infected tick. Since Lyme disease has occurred in more than 40 states, everyone should take steps to protect against it.

Not all ticks carry Lyme disease. Lyme disease is spread mainly by a tick that attaches itself to field mice and deer. It is sometimes called a deer tick and is found around beaches and in wooded and grassy areas. Like all ticks, it attaches itself to any warm-blooded animal that brushes by, including humans.

Deer ticks are small and difficult to see. They can be as small as a poppy seed. Adult deer ticks are only as large as a grape seed.

The risk for getting Lyme disease from the bite of an infected tick exists at any time of year, but in the northern states the risk is greatest between May and late August.

Signals of Lyme Disease

The first signal of Lyme disease is usually a rash at the bite site. It may appear within days or weeks of the bite. It may spread up to 5 to 7 inches across. In fair-skinned people, the center is lighter than the outer edges, which are red and raised. In dark-skinned people, the area may look black and blue, like a bruise. Other signals of Lyme disease include fever, headache, weakness, and joint and muscle pain similar to the pain of "flu." The signals may not all appear at the same time. You can have Lyme disease without developing a rash.

In its later stages Lyme disease may cause arthritis, numbness, memory loss, problems seeing or hearing, high fever, and stiff neck.

First Aid for Bites and Stings

If you find a tick, grasp it with fine-tipped tweezers, as close to the skin as possible, and pull slowly and firmly. Use a glove, plastic wrap, a piece of paper, or a leaf to protect your fingers if you do not have tweezers. If you use your bare fingers, wash your hands immediately. Do not try to burn a tick off with a hot match or a burning cigarette. Do not coat the tick with petroleum jelly or nail polish or prick it with a pin.

If you cannot remove the tick, or if its mouthparts stay in your skin, get medical care. Once the tick is removed, wash the area with soap and water. Apply an antibiotic ointment if it is available. Look at the area of the bite periodically. If you see a rash or develop flu-like symptoms, seek medical help immediately.

To care for an insect sting, first look to see if the stinger is in the skin. If it is, try to remove it. Scrape the stinger away from the skin with your fingernail or a plastic card such as a credit card. Do not use tweezers to remove the stinger. Next, wash the site with soap and water and cover it to keep it clean. Put a cold pack on the area that has been stung to reduce swelling and pain. Place a cloth between the skin and the cold pack to prevent skin damage.

Signals of Allergic Reaction

Allergic reaction usually occurs within seconds or minutes of the bite. The area that was bitten or stung usually swells and turns red. Other signals include hives, itching, rash, weakness, nausea, vomiting, and dizziness. The victim may have breathing difficulty. He or she may cough or wheeze.

First Aid for Allergic Reaction

If you see any of the signals of allergic reaction after someone has been bitten or stung, watch the person carefully. If the person has any trouble breathing or says that his or her throat is closing, call EMS at once. Help him or her into the most comfortable position for breathing. Monitor the ABCs and reassure the victim.

People who know they are very allergic to certain substances usually try to avoid them. They may carry a special kit in case they have a severe allergic reaction.

SNAKEBITES

Of the 8,000 people bitten by snakes annually in the United States, fewer than 12 die. Most deaths occur because the victim has an allergic reaction or weakened body system, or because much time passes before the victim receives medical care.

Elaborate care for snakebite is usually unnecessary because in most cases the victim can reach professional medical care within 30 minutes. Care can often be reached much faster, since most bites occur near the home, not in the wild.

First Aid for Snakebite

Call EMS for a victim of snakebite. Wash the wound and keep the affected part still. Splint a bitten arm or leg. Keep the affected area lower than the heart to slow down the progress of the venom from the bite site to the heart. If possible, carry a victim who must be transported, or have him or her walk slowly.

If you know the victim cannot get professional medical care within 30 minutes, consider suctioning the wound using a snakebite kit. People at risk of snakebites in the wild (away from medical care) should carry a snakebite kit and know how to use its contents.

Commonly Asked Questions About Bites

1. **Q.** Is it a good idea to put a cold pack on a snakebite?
    A. No. Medical experts in the past suggested that cooling the bitten area would slow the spread of venom. More recently, however, it has been found out that venom is not affected by cold. In addition, applying ice improperly can freeze the tissue.
2. **Q.** Should a person bitten by a snake be given aspirin to relieve pain?
    A. No. Do not give aspirin, since it widens (dilates) the blood vessels, which will circulate venom in the body faster.

Human and Animal Bites

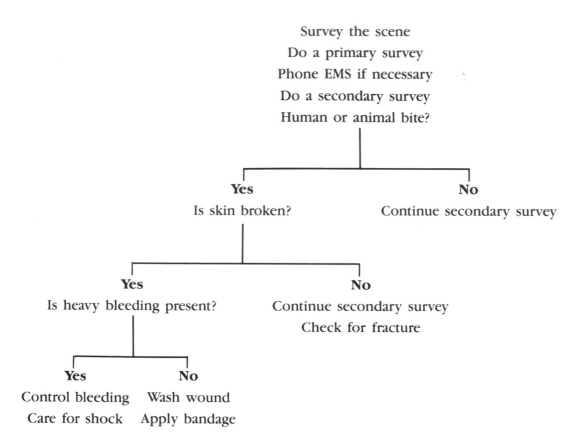

Survey the scene
Do a primary survey
Phone EMS if necessary
Do a secondary survey
Human or animal bite?

Yes   **No**
Is skin broken?   Continue secondary survey

Yes   **No**
Is heavy bleeding present?   Continue secondary survey
                                                Check for fracture

Yes   **No**
Control bleeding   Wash wound
Care for shock   Apply bandage

In the case of an animal bite, the animal needs to be captured for observation to check for rabies. Do not attempt to do this yourself. The proper authorities, such as the police and animal control, will try to capture the animal to observe it for rabies.

Insect Bites and Stings

Survey the scene
Do a primary survey
Phone EMS if allergic reaction
Do a secondary survey
Insect bite or sting?

Yes

Scrape off stinger with object like
a credit card or remove insect with
tweezers

Wash well with soap and water

Cover affected area with dressing
and apply cold pack

If allergic reaction, care for shock

Monitor ABCs

No

Continue secondary survey

Signals of allergic reaction include: pain, swelling of the
throat, redness or discoloration at the site, itching, hives,
decreased consciousness, or difficult or noisy breathing.

Snakebites

Survey the scene

Do a primary survey

Phone EMS
(or transport if EMS is more than 30 minutes away)

Do a secondary survey

Snakebite?

Yes

Keep victim calm

Wash wound

If bite on arm or leg, keep bitten area below
the level of the heart and splint

Care for shock

Monitor ABCs

No

Continue secondary survey

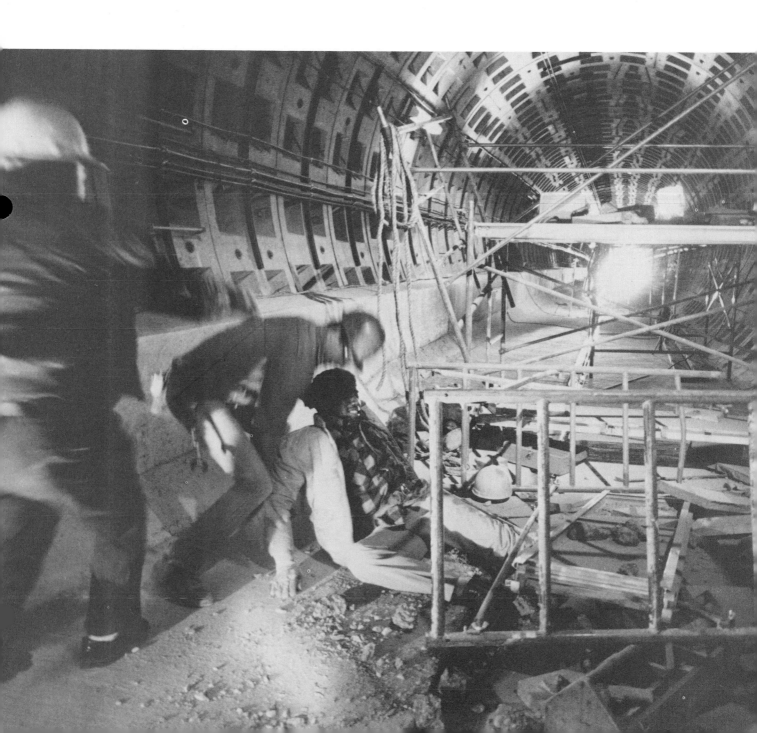

Learning Objectives

In this unit you will learn how to—
1. *Care for:*
   - *Fractures.*
   - *Dislocations.*
   - *Sprains.*
   - *Strains.*
2. *Splint the following:*
   - *The forearm.*
   - *The leg.*
   - *The ankle.*

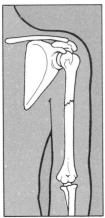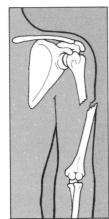

Figure 38
Closed Fracture (left); Open Fracture (right)

Fractures, dislocations, sprains, and strains are injuries that occur to the musculoskeletal system. The musculoskeletal system consists of the bones, muscles, ligaments, and tendons.

FRACTURES

Definition

Fractures are breaks or cracks in bones. They are defined as either closed or open *(Fig. 38).* Closed fractures leave the skin unbroken. They are more common than open fractures. An open fracture involves an open wound. Open fractures are more serious than closed fractures because of the risks of infection and severe bleeding. Fracture of a large bone can cause severe shock because bones and soft tissue may bleed heavily.

Fractures can be accompanied by internal injuries. For example, victims with fractured ribs can also have injuries to the lungs, kidneys, or liver.

Common Causes

Fractures can be caused by motor-vehicle accidents, falls, sports injuries, or bone diseases. Ribs can be fractured when drivers are thrown against the steering wheel in motor-vehicle accidents.

DISLOCATIONS

Definition

A dislocation is an injury in which a bone is separated or displaced from its normal position at a joint. A dislocation may involve damage to the ligaments around the joint.

Common Causes

Dislocations can be caused by falls, sports injuries, and motor-vehicle accidents.

SPRAINS

Definition

A sprain is the partial or complete tearing of ligaments and other tissues at a joint. The more ligaments that are torn, the more severe the injury.

Common Causes

Like dislocations, sprains can be caused by falls, sports injuries, and motor-vehicle accidents.

STRAINS

Definition

A strain is a stretching and tearing of muscle or tendon fibers. It is sometimes called a "muscle pull" or "tear."

Common Causes

Strains are often caused by lifing something improperly or lifting something too heavy. They often occur in the neck or back. Strains of the neck or lower back can be very painful.

Signals of Fractures, Dislocations, Sprains, and Strains

The signals of these injuries are very similar. Five common signals of musculoskeletal injuries are pain, swelling, deformity, discoloration or bruising of the skin, and inability to use the affected part normally.

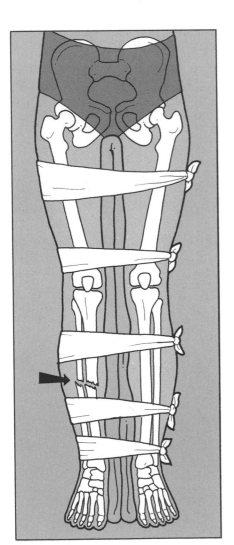

Figure 39
Leg Splint

First Aid for Fractures, Dislocations, Sprains, and Strains

Sometimes it is difficult to tell whether an injury is a fracture, dislocation, sprain, or strain. Since you cannot be sure which of these a victim might have, always care for it as a fracture. If EMS is on the way, do not move the victim. Control any bleeding first. Care for shock, and monitor ABCs. If you are going to transport the victim to a medical facility, follow this general rule: "When in doubt, splint."

Splinting is a process of immobilizing a suspected fracture. Materials that can immobilize a fractured bone and the joints above and below it can be used to splint. (Examples are rolled-up newspapers, magazines, and pieces of wood.) Commercial splints are also available.

The purposes of splinting are—
- To immobilize a possibly fractured part of the body.
- To lessen pain.
- To prevent further damage to soft tissues.
- To reduce the risk of serious bleeding.
- To reduce the possibility of loss of circulation in the injured part.
- To prevent closed fractures from becoming open fractures.

The basic principles of splinting are—
- Splint only if you can do it without causing more pain and discomfort to the victim.
- Splint an injury in the position you find it.
- Apply the splint so that it immobilizes the fractured bone and the joints above and below the fracture.
- Check circulation before and after splinting.

If there are no splinting supplies available, splint the broken part of the body to another part. For example, a broken arm can be splinted to the chest. A fractured leg can be splinted to the other, uninjured leg *(Fig. 39)*.

If the injury is a closed fracture, dislocation, sprain, or strain, apply a cold pack. Do not apply a cold pack to an open fracture. This would require you to put pressure on the wound and may cause discomfort to the victim.

Next, elevate the injured area. Do not attempt to elevate a part you suspect is fractured until it has been splinted.

For any of these injuries, care for shock and monitor ABCs.

Head, Neck, and Back Injuries

Injury of the head, neck, and back (spinal injury) is serious and difficult to care for. Think about these injuries as possibilities when caring for a victim who has suffered **traumatic injury.** Examples of situations in which traumatic injury may occur are falls, motor-vehicle accidents, and diving or other sports-related accidents.

If the victim has an obvious head injury, suspect the possibility of spinal cord injury also. If the victim is unconscious and your survey of the scene suggests traumatic injury to the head, care for him or her as if there is a spinal injury.

If you do suspect a spinal injury, stabilize the victim's head and neck as you found them by placing your hands along both sides of the head *(Fig. 40).* This keeps the head in line with the spine and prevents movement.

If you must move the victim, do it carefully, using the clothes drag rescue method (pages 154–155).

Stay with the victim and continue to stabilize the head and neck until EMS arrives. Monitor ABCs.

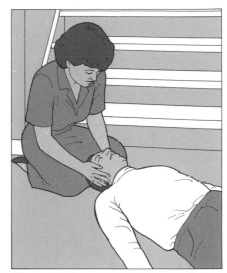

Figure 40
In-line Stabilization

Skill Sheets: Splinting

How to Use a Rigid Splint and Sling

You are doing a secondary survey and suspect that the victim may have a closed fracture of the forearm.

☐ ☐ **Splint**

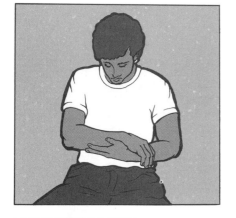

If possible, have the victim support fractured arm in front of body.

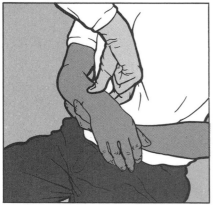

Check radial pulse on fractured arm.

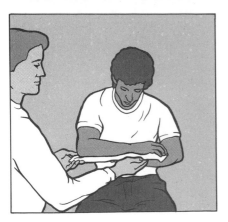

Place splint under fractured forearm. Have victim or bystander hold splint in place if possible.

Place a soft object (for example, a roll of gauze) in palm of victim's hand to keep hand in its natural position.

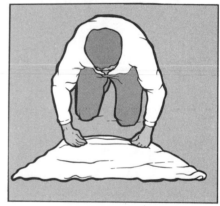

Fold 2 triangular bandages: Start at the point and fold toward the wider end.

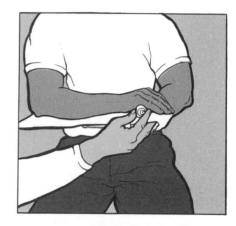

Thread the 2 bandages under splint, 1 above and the other below the fracture.

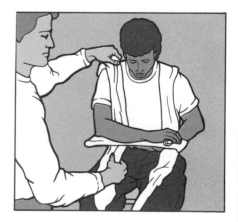

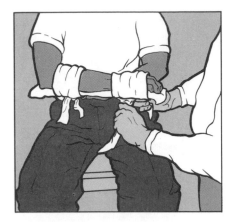

Tie ends of each bandage together on underside of splint, leaving fractured area uncovered.

Splint should be snug but not so tight that it constricts blood flow to wrist.

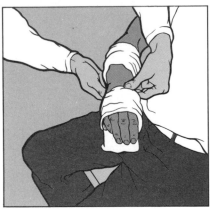

Check radial pulse and look at fingertips to be sure bandages are not too tight. (Fingertips would look bluish.)

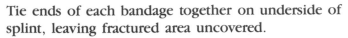

☐ ☐ **Sling**

Open a triangular bandage and thread one end under injured arm so that it goes across victim's chest and over uninjured shoulder.

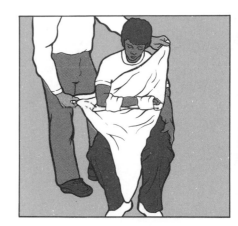

Bring other end of bandage over fractured arm, across chest, and over opposite shoulder. Point of sling should now rest behind elbow. Victim's hand should be raised about 4 inches above elbow and fingertips should be exposed.

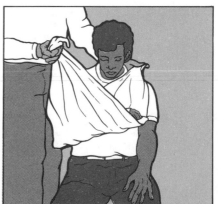

Tie ends of triangular bandage at side of neck. Place a pad under the knot.

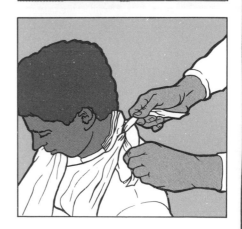

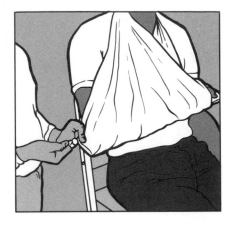

Tie or pin the point of sling at elbow if possible.

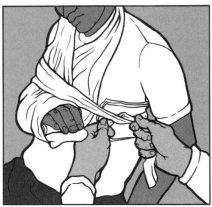

☐ ☐ **Binder**

Use another folded triangular bandage to bind the sling. Tie ends together on opposite side under uninjured arm. Place a pad under knot.

How to Use Another Body Part to Splint a Fracture (Anatomic Splint)

You are doing a secondary survey and suspect that the victim may have a closed fracture of the leg.

Partner Check
Instructor Check

☐ ☐ **Leg splint**

Thread 5 folded triangular bandages under legs: 1 each at ankles, at lower legs, below knees, above knees, and at thighs. Leave fracture exposed. Do not cover with bandage.

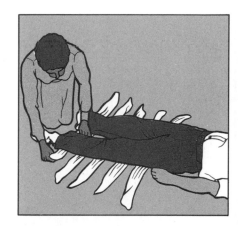

Place padding (blanket or pillow) between legs.

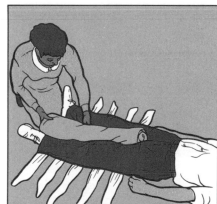

Tie ends of each bandage together, with knots on uninjured leg.

Check to see that bandages are snug but not too tight. You should be able to fit only 1 finger under the bandage.

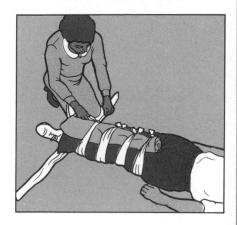

119

How to Use a Soft Splint

You are doing a secondary survey and suspect that the victim may have a closed fracture of the ankle.

Partner Check
Instructor Check

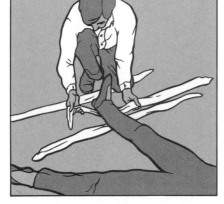

☐ ☐ **Ankle splint**

Leave footwear in place (sock or shoe).

Thread 2 folded triangular bandages under ankle and lower leg.

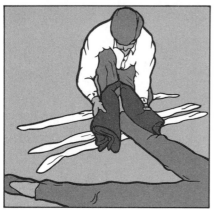

Fold or wrap blanket or pillow gently around ankle.

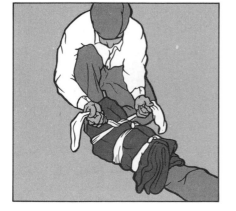

Firmly tie blanket or pillow in place around ankle and lower leg with 2 bandages.

Tie a third bandage around the foot.

Check to see that bandages are snug but not too tight.

Final Instructor Check _____

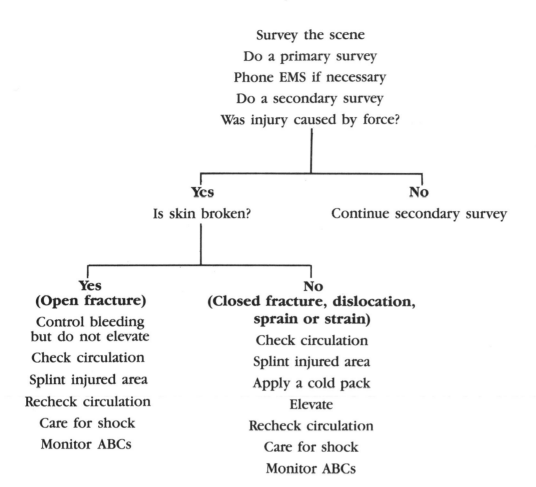

Survey the scene
Do a primary survey
Phone EMS if necessary
Do a secondary survey
Was injury caused by force?

Yes — Is skin broken?

No — Continue secondary survey

Yes (Open fracture)
Control bleeding but do not elevate
Check circulation
Splint injured area
Recheck circulation
Care for shock
Monitor ABCs

No (Closed fracture, dislocation, sprain or strain)
Check circulation
Splint injured area
Apply a cold pack
Elevate
Recheck circulation
Care for shock
Monitor ABCs

Sometimes a forceful blow can cause a head, neck, or back injury. Signals of these injuries can include any or all of these: pain and swelling, changes in level of consciousness, blood or clear fluid draining from the nose or ears, bruising under the eyes or behind the ears, loss of feeling in hands or feet, and an inability to move hands or feet. If you suspect a head, neck, or back injury, do not move the victim or stop the flow of blood or clear fluids coming from the nose or ears.

11

Poisoning

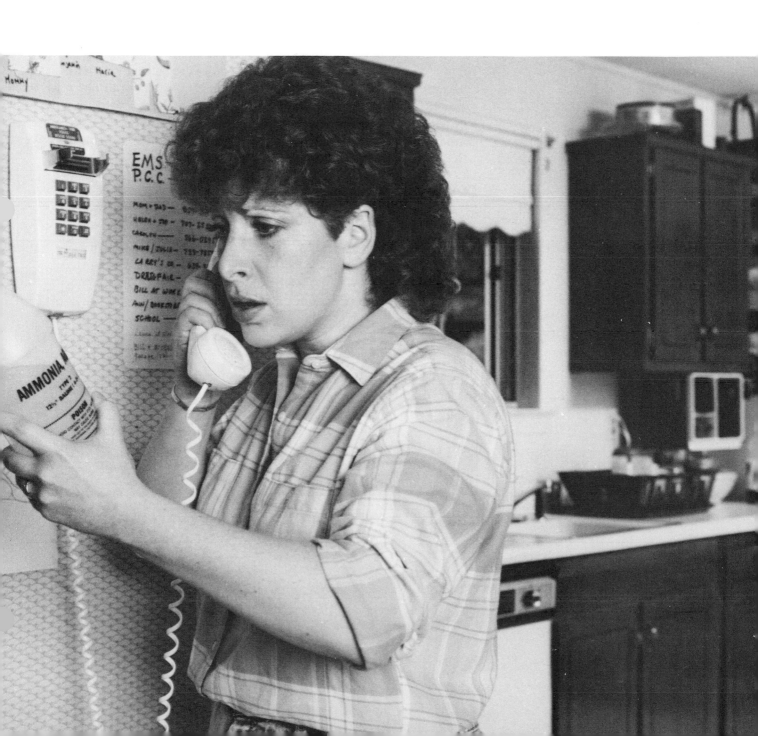

Poisoning

Learning Objectives

In this unit you will learn how to care for a victim who has—
1. Swallowed poison.
2. Inhaled poison.
3. Absorbed poison.

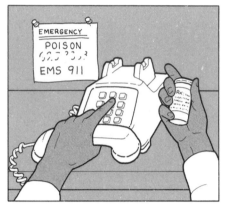

Figure 41
Phone Poison Control Center

It is estimated that between 1 and 2 million poisonings occur each year in the United States. More than 90 percent of all poisonings take place in the home. Most poisonings happen to children under the age of 5 years, but less than 5 percent of them die. Poisoning deaths among adults 18 and older has markedly increased in the last 30 years.

A poisoning presents problems for the lay public as well as EMS personnel. Some poisons are quick-acting, with characteristic signals. Others act slowly, and cannot be easily identified. Sometimes you may be able to identify the poison, sometimes not. **The most important thing is to recognize that a poisoning may have occurred.**

A network of Poison Control Centers (PCCs) exists to help people deal with poisonings. These centers are staffed by medical professionals who will tell you what care to give. You should post your local PCC number by your phone *(Fig. 41)*. If you do not know your PCC number, call your local emergency number immediately.

Definition

A poison is any substance—solid, liquid, or gas—that causes injury or death when introduced into the body. There are four main ways a person can be poisoned: by swallowing, by inhaling, by absorbing through the skin, and by injecting *(Fig. 42)*.

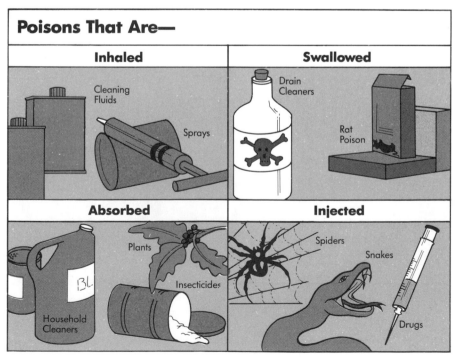

Figure 42
Poisons

124

SWALLOWED POISON

Common Causes

The most common circumstances in which people swallow poison are taking overdoses of medicine, taking drugs with alcohol, putting cleaning products and other chemicals in unlabeled food containers, and being careless. Young children risk poisoning when medicines, plants, and household products are within their reach.

Signals

A person who has swallowed poison may have any or all of these signals: nausea, vomiting, diarrhea, chest or abdominal pain, breathing difficulty, sweating, loss of consciousness, and seizures. Other signals are burn injuries around the mouth or on the tongue, evidence of opened or spilled containers, and overturned or damaged plants.

If you think the person may be poisoned, call the Poison Control Center or EMS immediately.

First Aid

For first aid, quickly take any containers to the phone; then call EMS and the local Poison Control Center and follow their instructions. Care for shock and check breathing frequently. Do not give anything by mouth until you have been advised by medical professionals.

Be sure to save any containers and vomit for EMS. These will help them identify the poison and give the appropriate treatment.

INHALED POISON

Common Causes

Sources of inhaled poisoning can include carbon monoxide (from car exhaust, defective cooking equipment, fire, and charcoal grills), carbon dioxide (from wells and sewers), smoke, refrigeration gases, fumes from spray chemicals, and industrial and home chemicals.

Signals

The signals of inhaled poisoning can include any or all of the following: dizziness, headache, breathing difficulty, unconsciousness, and pale or bluish skin color.

First Aid

You must not put yourself in danger. Unless you are trained to enter a scene in which poisonous gases are present and have the proper equipment, you should not try to rescue a victim. Call EMS, and stay clear of danger.

If you can reach the victim, remove him or her from the poisonous environment. Get to fresh air. Check ABCs. Call EMS and the Poison Control Center and follow their instructions. Monitor ABCs.

If you work around poisonous chemicals, you should know first aid procedures specific to them. Also, be familiar with available emergency equipment such as masks; know where the equipment is kept and how to use it. Be sure that your work area is properly ventilated.

ABSORBED POISON

Common Causes

Many absorbed poisons are corrosives or irritants that injure the skin and are then taken into body tissues. People can be poisoned by insecticides; agricultural, lawn, and garden chemicals; plants such as poison ivy, oak, or sumac; and venom from certain marine life.

Signals

The signals of absorbed poisoning include any or all of the following: skin reactions, itching, eye irritation, changes in breathing and pulse, and headache.

First Aid

Care for a victim of absorbed poisoning includes removing the victim from the source of the poison, flushing all affected areas with lots of water, removing clothes with the poison on them, and caring for shock. Monitor ABCs.

INJECTED POISON

Sources of injected poisons are stings from insects and venomous marine life, spider bites, snakebites, and drugs injected by needles. A small percentage of people stung or bitten will have an allergic reaction to the venom.

Care for injected poisons (other than injected drugs) is found in the unit on bites and stings.

Commonly Asked Questions About Poisoning

1. **Q.** Shouldn't I first dilute a swallowed poison before calling the Poison Control Center?

   A. No. In the case of some medications, for example, diluting them causes them to dissolve and be absorbed by the victim's body faster. Before diluting a poison, call EMS or the Poison Control Center quickly and follow their advice.

2. **Q.** What should I have on hand as first aid supplies for poisoning?

   A. Keep the following on hand: syrup of ipecac and activated charcoal. Syrup of ipecac induces vomiting, and activated charcoal can bind or neutralize certain poisons. Do not use these without the advice of a Poison Control Center.

3. **Q.** Is it true that victims of carbon monoxide poisoning have "cherry red" lips and skin?

   A. No. The lips and skin of a victim of carbon monoxide poisoning are usually cyanotic, i.e., bluish in color. The "cherry red" color commonly associated with carbon monoxide poisoning most often occurs following death, and, therefore, is a poor indicator of carbon monoxide poisoning in a victim who is still alive.

Poisoning Action Guides

Swallowed Poison

Survey the scene

Do a primary survey

Do you suspect the victim swallowed poison?

Yes	No
Place victim on side if vomiting	Do a secondary survey
Phone EMS and the Poison Control Center; have containers in hand if possible	
Follow directions from EMS and the Poison Control Center	
Monitor ABCs	
Save containers and any vomit to give EMS	

Be Prepared for Poisoning Emergencies

1. Keep the number of the Poison Control Center near each phone. Fill out the list of emergency phone numbers at the end of this workbook, and put a copy by each phone. The Poison Control Center number for your community is ___1-800-682-9211___

2. Keep syrup of ipecac and activated charcoal on hand. Use these only when the Poison Control Center or other medical professionals instruct you to do so.

Inhaled Poison

Survey the scene
Is it safe for you to check victim?

Yes
Shout, "Help!"
Remove victim from source of poison
Get victim to fresh air
Do a primary survey
Place victim on side if vomiting
Phone EMS and Poison Control Center
Follow their directions
Monitor ABCs

No
Phone EMS
Stay clear of danger

Absorbed Poison

Survey the scene

Do a primary survey

Did victim come in contact with poison?

Yes	**No**
Remove victim from source of the poison	Do a secondary survey
Wash poison from skin	
Remove clothing and other articles with poison on them	
Phone EMS and the Poison Control Center	
Follow their directions	
Monitor ABCs	

12

Diabetic Emergencies

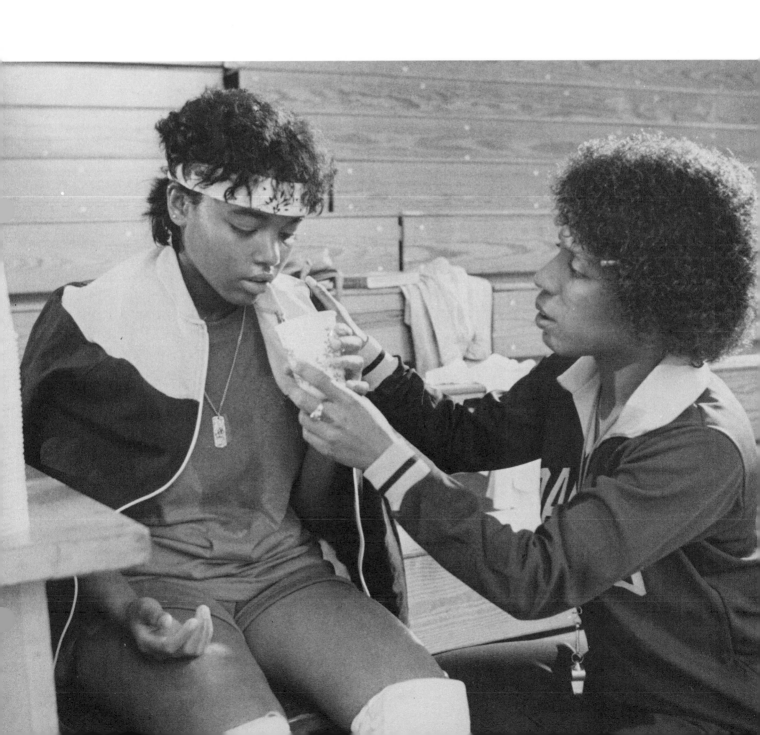

Diabetic Emergencies

Learning Objectives

In this unit you will learn how to care for the victim of a diabetic emergency.

Definition

To maintain life, blood carries sugar as nourishment for body cells. Insulin is a hormone that helps the body to use the sugar. When enough insulin is not available, body cells do not get enough nourishment, and diabetes results. People with diabetes keep their condition under control by taking medication and regulating their diet and activity. In diabetes, two very different emergencies can arise: insulin reaction (insulin shock) and diabetic coma.

Insulin reaction occurs when too much insulin is in the body. Too much insulin rapidly reduces the level of sugar in the blood, and brain cells suffer. Insulin reaction can be caused by taking too much medication, by failing to eat, by heavy exercise, and by emotional factors.

Diabetic coma happens when there is too much sugar and too little insulin in the blood, and body cells do not get enough nourishment. Diabetic coma can be caused by eating too much sugar, by not taking prescribed medication, by stress, and by infection.

Signals

The major signals of insulin reaction and diabetic coma are the same. They include changes in the level of consciousness, including dizziness, drowsiness, and confusion; rapid breathing; rapid pulse; and feeling and looking ill.

The basic care for insulin reaction and diabetic coma is the same. You do not have to decide which condition the person has.

First Aid for Diabetic Emergencies

First, do a primary survey and care for any life-threatening conditions. Do a secondary survey if the victim is conscious. Ask the victim if he or she is a diabetic or look for a medical alert tag. If the person tells you he or she is a diabetic and shows any of the signals listed on page 132, then you should suspect a diabetic emergency.

If the person is conscious and can take food or fluids, give him or her sugar. Most candy, fruit juices, and nondiet soft drinks have enough sugar to be effective. You can also give table sugar, either dry or dissolved in a glass of water. The sugar will quickly help someone who has too much insulin in the blood, and will not harm a person with too little insulin in the blood. Often diabetics know what is wrong and will ask for something with sugar in it. They may carry sugar for these occasions. If the person does not feel better within about 5 minutes after taking sugar, call EMS.

If the person is unconscious, do not give anything by mouth. Call EMS, monitor the ABCs, and maintain normal body temperature.

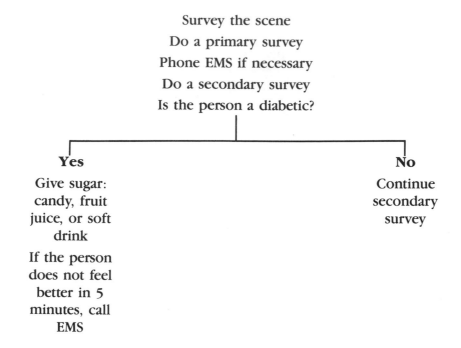

Survey the scene
Do a primary survey
Phone EMS if necessary
Do a secondary survey
Is the person a diabetic?

Yes

Give sugar: candy, fruit juice, or soft drink

If the person does not feel better in 5 minutes, call EMS

No

Continue secondary survey

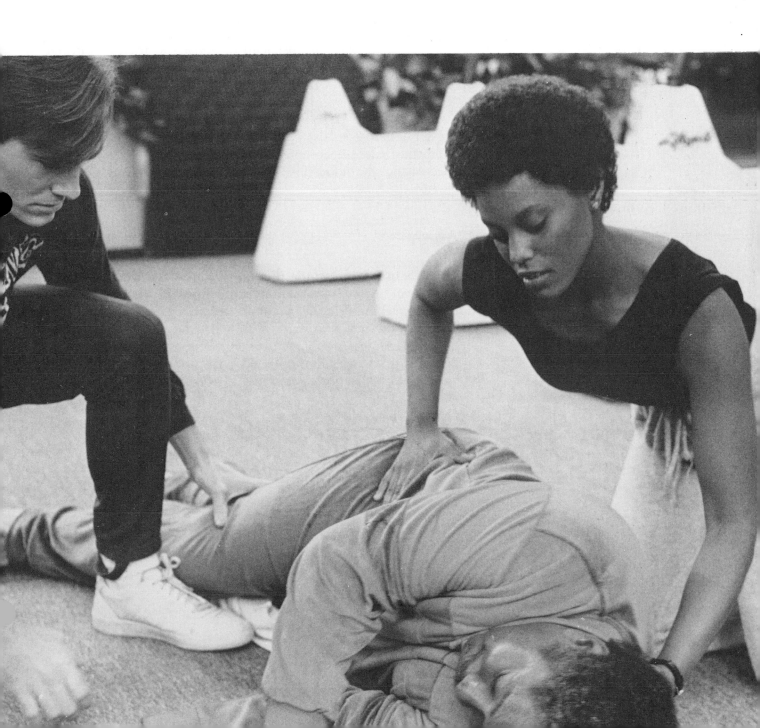

Learning Objective

In this unit you will learn how to care for a victim of a stroke.

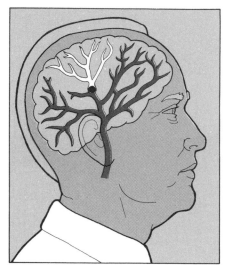

Figure 43
Blood Clot in Brain

Definition

A stroke is a condition that occurs when the blood flow to the brain is interrupted long enough to cause damage. People over age 50 are the most common victims, but younger people can have them, too.

Common Causes

There are three causes of stroke:
1. The most common cause is a clot (thrombus or embolism) formed in an artery in the brain or carried to the brain in the bloodstream *(Fig. 43)*.
2. A second cause is a ruptured artery in the brain, resulting from a head injury, high blood pressure, a weak spot in the wall of a blood vessel (aneurysm), or fat deposits lining a vessel (atherosclerosis).
3. The third cause is compression of an artery in the brain, decreasing the blood flow. This is often the result of a brain tumor.

Signals

The signals of stroke include sudden weakness and numbness of the face, arm, or leg, often on one side only. The victim may have difficulty speaking or understanding speech. Vision may be blurred or dimmed; the pupils of the eyes may be of unequal size. Other signals are dizziness; confusion; sudden, severe headache; ringing in the ears; or changes in mood. The victim may become unconscious or lose bowel or bladder control.

First Aid

If the victim is unconscious, make sure he or she has an open airway, and care for any life-threatening conditions. If the victim vomits, place him or her on one side so that any fluids can drain from the mouth *(Fig. 44)*. If necessary, use your finger to sweep some of the material from the mouth. Call EMS immediately. Stay with the victim, and monitor ABCs.

If the victim is conscious, do a secondary survey. If signals of stroke are present, phone EMS. Reassure the victim. Often he or she does not understand what has happened. Help the victim rest in the most comfortable position. Do not give anything to eat or drink. If the victim is drooling or having difficulty swallowing, place him or her on one side to help drain any fluids or vomitus from the mouth. Monitor ABCs.

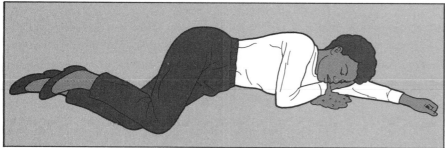

Figure 44
Position for Stroke Victim Who Is Vomiting

Survey the scene
Do a primary survey
Is victim conscious?

Yes

Do a secondary survey
If signals of stroke are present:
Phone EMS

Help victim rest in most
comfortable position

Do not give anything by mouth

Monitor ABCs

If victim vomits, place him or her
on side

Reassure victim

No

Phone EMS
Monitor ABCs

If victim vomits, place him
or her on side

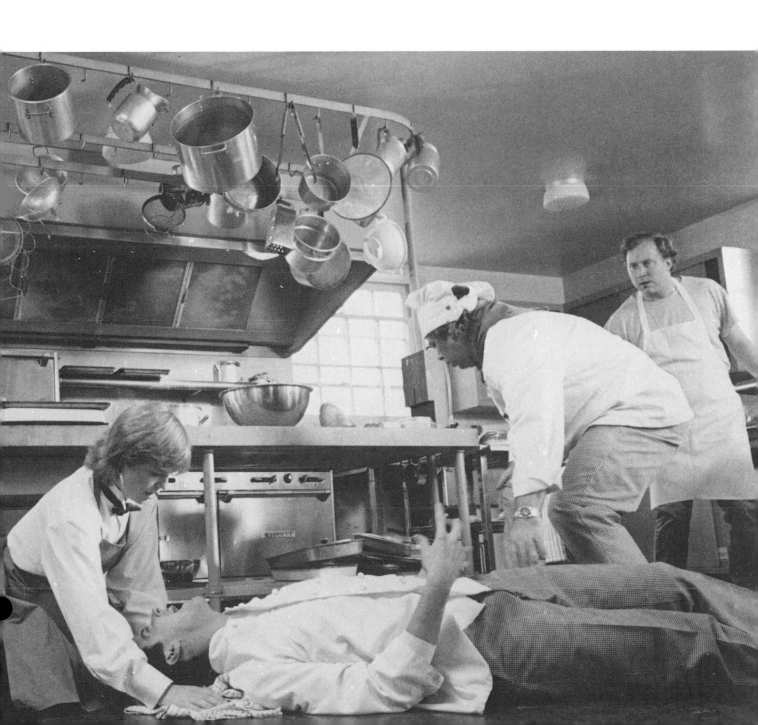

Learning Objective

In this unit you will learn how to care for a victim of a seizure.

Common Causes

Seizures may be caused by an acute condition such as head injury, disease, fever, or infection. They may also be caused by a condition called epilepsy. Epilepsy is usually controlled with medication, but some people with epilepsy still have seizures from time to time.

Signals

Some people have an aura before the onset of a seizure. An aura is an unusual sensation or feeling, such as a visual hallucination; a strange sound, taste, or smell; or a sense of urgency to move to safety. The person may have time to tell bystanders and sit down before the seizure begins.

Seizures can range from mild blackouts to sudden, uncontrolled muscle contractions called convulsions. The mild blackouts might be mistaken for daydreaming. The convulsions might last for several minutes.

First Aid

If you know the person has epilepsy, it is usually not necessary to call EMS unless—
- The seizure lasts longer than a few minutes.
- Another seizure begins soon after the first.
- He or she does not regain consciousness after the jerking movements have stopped.

However, you should call EMS when someone having a seizure also—
- Is pregnant.
- Is known to be a diabetic.
- Appears to be injured.
- Is in water.

A person having a seizure cannot control it. Do not hold or restrain the person. This can cause musculoskeletal injuries. Do not try to put anything between the teeth. You should protect the victim from injury, and keep his or her airway open. You can prevent injuries by moving anything that is nearby and might get in the way, such as furniture or equipment *(Fig. 45)*. Protect the head by placing a thin cushion, such as folded clothing, beneath it. If the victim vomits, roll him or her on one side.

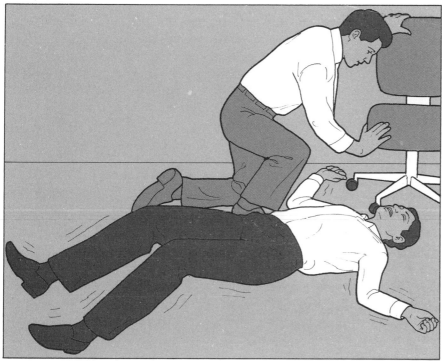

Figure 45
Preventing Injuries by Clearing Area

When the seizure is over, the person will be drowsy and disoriented and will need to rest. Do a secondary survey to check for injuries. Reassure the person. Stay with the person until he or she is fully conscious and aware of the surroundings.

Survey the scene

Do a primary survey

Phone EMS if necessary

Do a secondary survey

Is the victim having a convulsive seizure?

Yes

Protect victim from injury, but
do not restrain

Do not place anything between
victim's teeth

Place thin cushion beneath
victim's head

If victim vomits, roll him or
her on one side

When seizure is over, check ABCs

Do a secondary survey

Reassure victim

No

Continue secondary survey

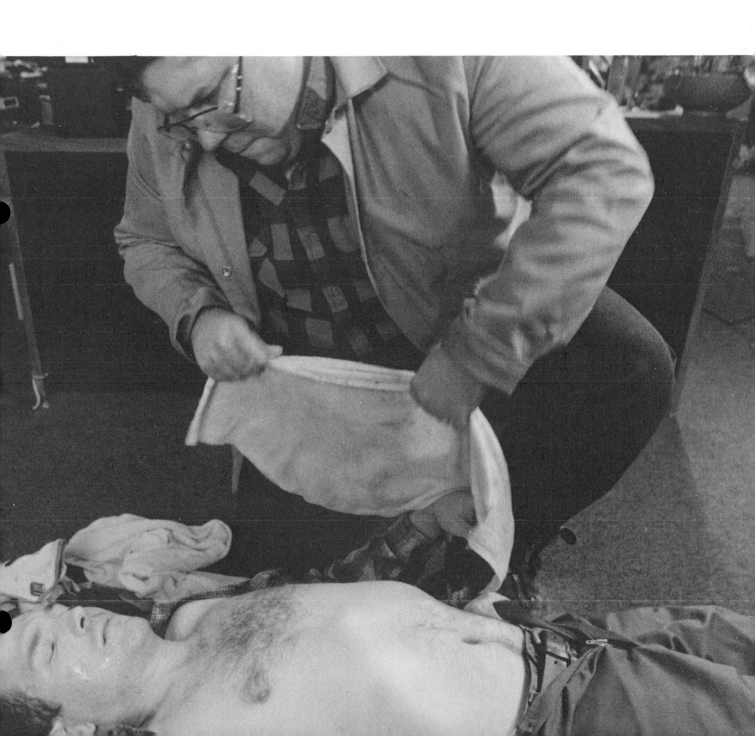

HEAT EMERGENCIES

On hot, humid days with no breeze, anyone may be affected by the heat. People who are especially susceptible to extreme heat are the very young and the very old, the chronically ill, the overweight, those who work in hot places, and athletes. They may suffer heat stroke, heat exhaustion *(Fig. 46),* or heat cramps.

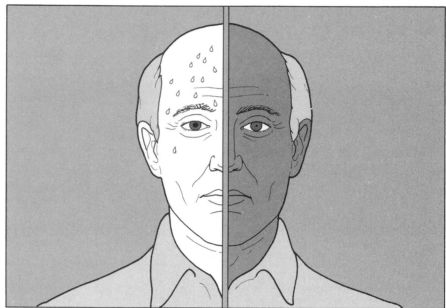

Figure 46
Heat Exhaustion (left); Heat Stroke (right)

Heat Stroke

Heat stroke is life-threatening. The victim's temperature-control system, which produces sweating to cool the body, stops working. The body temperature can rise so high that brain damage and death may result if the body is not cooled quickly. Help must be fast. Quickly cool the victim's body. Heat stroke requires medical attention.

Signals
Signals of heat stroke are dry, hot, red skin; very high body temperature—sometimes as high as 106 degrees; progressive loss of consciousness; fast, weak pulse; and fast, shallow breathing.

First Aid

Heat stroke is a life-threatening situation. Call EMS. Get the person out of the heat and into a cooler place. Cool the victim fast. Immerse him or her in a cool bath, or wrap wet sheets around the body and fan it. Care for shock while waiting for EMS to arrive. If the victim is conscious, offer cool water to drink. Do not let the victim drink too quickly. Give one-half glass (4 ounces) about every 15 minutes.

Heat Exhaustion

Heat exhaustion is less dangerous than heat stroke. It typically occurs when people exercise heavily or work in a warm, humid place where body fluids are lost through heavy sweating. Fluid loss causes blood flow to decrease in the vital organs, resulting in a form of shock.

Signals

The usual signals of heat exhaustion are cool, moist, pale, or red skin; heavy sweating; dilated pupils; headache; nausea; dizziness and weakness; and exhaustion. Body temperature will be normal or below normal.

First Aid

Get the person out of the heat and into a cooler place. Place him or her on the back, with feet up. Either remove or loosen the victim's clothing. Cool him or her by fanning and applying cold packs (putting a cloth between the pack and the victim's skin) or wet towels or sheets. Care for shock. Give the victim one-half glassful of water to drink every 15 minutes, if he or she is fully conscious and can tolerate it. Without prompt care, heat exhaustion can quickly become heat stroke.

Heat Cramps

Heat cramps are muscular pains and spasms due to heavy exertion. They usually involve the abdominal muscles or legs. It is generally thought that the loss of water and salt from heavy sweating causes the cramps.

First Aid

As with other heat emergencies, get the person to a cooler place. If the victim has no other injuries and can tolerate water, give him or her one-half glassful every 15 minutes for an hour. Lightly stretch the muscle and gently massage the area. Watch the victim carefully after he or she begins to feel better.

COLD EMERGENCIES

On days with low temperatures, high winds, and humidity, anyone can suffer from the extreme cold. Severe cold exposure can be life-threatening. Several factors increase the harmful effects of cold: being very young or very old, wet clothing, having wounds or fractures, smoking, drinking alcoholic beverages, fatigue, emotional stress, and certain diseases and medications. People exposed to severe cold can suffer from hypothermia or frostbite.

Hypothermia

Signals

The signals of hypothermia include shivering, dizziness, numbness, confusion, weakness, impaired judgement, impaired vision, and drowsiness *(Fig. 47)*. The stages are—

1. Shivering.
2. Apathy.
3. Loss of consciousness.
4. Decreasing pulse rate and breathing rate.
5. Death.

   As hypothermia progresses, the victim may move clumsily and have trouble holding things. In the later stages, he or she may stop shivering.

First Aid

As the action guide shows, call EMS. You should get a victim of hypothermia out of the cold and into dry clothing. Warm up his or her body slowly. Give nothing to eat or drink unless the victim is fully conscious. Monitor ABCs.

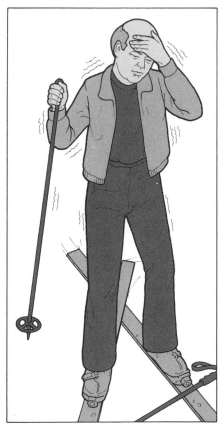

Figure 47
Hypothermia

146

Frostbite

Frostbite is the most common injury caused by exposure to cold. It happens when ice crystals form in body tissues, usually the nose, ears, chin, cheeks, fingers, or toes. This restricts blood flow to the injured parts. The effect is worse if the frostbitten parts are thawed and then refrozen.

Signals

The first sign of frostbite may be that the skin is slightly flushed. The skin color of the frostbitten area then changes to white or grayish yellow and finally grayish blue, as the frostbite develops. Pain is sometimes felt early on but later goes away. The frostbitten part feels very cold and numb. The victim may not be aware of the injury.

Frostbite has degrees of tissue damage. Mild frostbite looks white or grayish, and the skin feels hard, even though the underlying tissue feels soft *(Fig. 48)*. In moderate frostbite, large blisters form on the surface and in the tissues underneath *(Fig. 49)*. The frostbitten area is hard, cold, and insensitive. If freezing is deeper than the skin, tissue damage is severe *(Fig. 50)*. **Gangrene** may result from the loss of blood supply to the area.

First Aid

Get the victim into a warm place. Put the frozen parts in warm (100–105 degrees) but not hot water. Handle them gently, and do not rub or massage them. If the toes or fingers are affected, put dry, sterile gauze between them after warming them. Loosely bandage the injured parts. If the part has been thawed and refrozen, then you should rewarm it at room temperature.

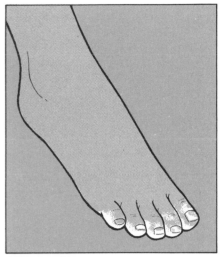

Figure 48
Mild Frostbite

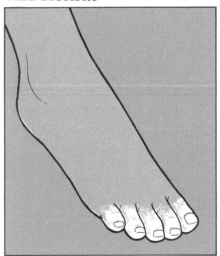

Figure 49
Moderate Frostbite

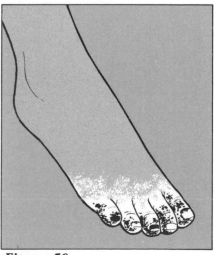

Figure 50
Severe Frostbite

Commonly Asked Questions About Temperature Extremes

1. **Q.** Is it a good idea to give aspirin to someone who is suffering from extreme heat?

   A. No. Aspirin does not lower the fever that results from heat exposure. Also, since the victim is usually dehydrated, the concentration of the aspirin would be higher than usual and could poison the victim.

2. **Q.** Is it a good idea to give salt or electrolyte solutions to someone who is suffering from extreme heat?

   A. Concentrated amounts of salt can cause nausea, which could lead to vomiting. Small sips of cool water should be given as long as the victim is fully conscious.

3. **Q.** Is it a good idea to rub a frostbitten part?

   A. Never rub a frostbitten part, since that can cause extensive tissue damage.

Heat Emergencies

Survey the scene
Do a primary survey
Phone EMS if necessary
Do a secondary survey
Was the victim exposed to heat?

Yes

Remove victim from heat
Have victim rest
Elevate feet
Loosen or remove clothing
Cool victim
If conscious, give ½ glass of water
about every 15 minutes, as tolerated

No

Continue secondary survey

Cold Emergencies

Survey the scene
Do a primary survey
Phone EMS if necesary
Do a secondary survey
Was the victim exposed to cold?

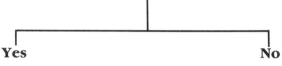

Yes   **No**

Remove from cold and get to warm place   Continue secondary survey

Remove any wet clothes and cover with
dry clothing or blankets

If conscious, give warm
fluids

Rewarm any frozen part
(such as fingers or toes) by
immersing in warm water

Do not give beverages containing alcohol or caffeine.
Give warm broth or water.

150

16 Rescues

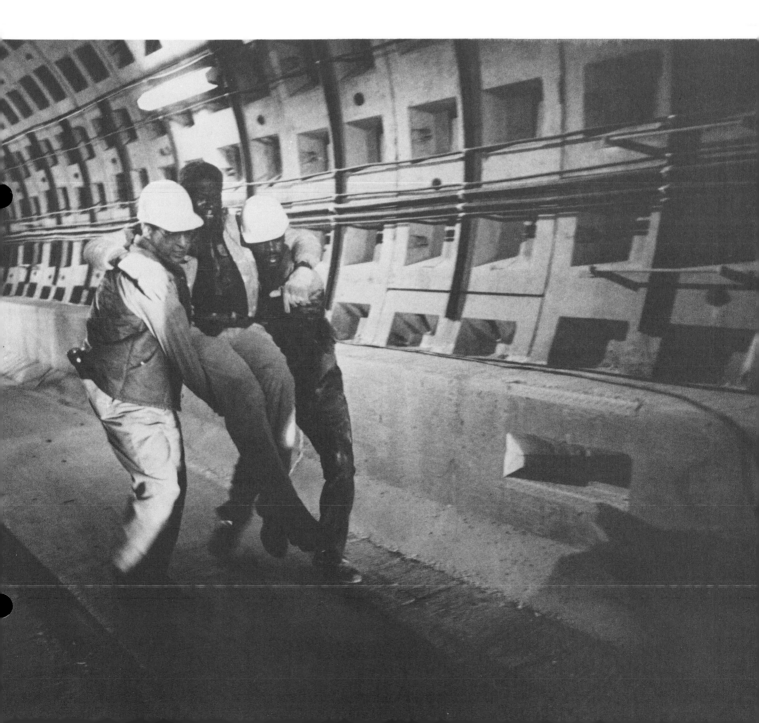

Learning Objectives

In this unit you will learn when it is appropriate to move a victim using the following methods:
1. Two-handed seat carry
2. Clothes drag
3. Foot drag

When There Is No Immediate Danger

If there is no immediate danger present, you should follow the emergency action principles and care for the victim at the scene while waiting for EMS to arrive. Your task is to give basic life support and keep injuries from getting worse. Moving a victim can make some injuries worse. For example, carelessly moving someone with a closed fracture could result in an open fracture. This would cause bleeding, possible nerve and muscle damage, and an increased chance of infection.

Remember: Unless it is absolutely necessary, do not move a victim. It is the role of EMS to move victims from the scene of the injury.

When There Is Immediate Danger

You should rescue or move a victim only if there is immediate danger to you and him or her. Immediate danger would be from fire, lack of oxygen, serious traffic hazard, risk of drowning, risk of explosion, exposure to bad weather, collapsing buildings, and electrical hazards. Being near a car that has been involved in an accident is not in itself dangerous. Cars rarely explode after accidents. However, you should always check to see that the car is in no danger of moving. Put on the parking brake and turn off the ignition if you can do these without moving the victim.

How to Move a Victim

If there is immediate danger and you must move a victim, remember to—

- Provide support for the victim's neck and spine.
- Avoid bending or twisting the victim.
- Drag a victim to safety, keeping the body straight. Never move it sideways.
- Lift from your knees, not with your back.

This unit gives three rescues to consider using when it becomes necessary to move a victim.

- If there is a second person who can help and you do not suspect a spinal injury, use the two-handed seat carry *(Fig. 51).*

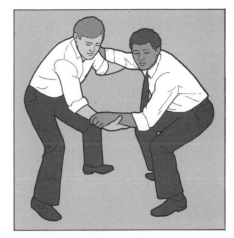

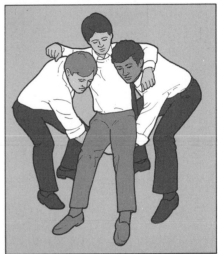

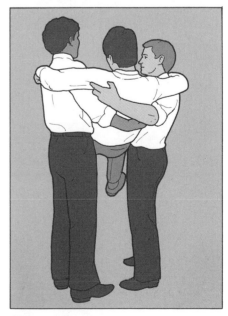

Figure 51
Two-Handed Seat Carry

• If you are alone and you suspect the victim might have a spinal injury, use the clothes drag *(Fig. 52)*. This allows you to give support to the victim's head while moving him or her.

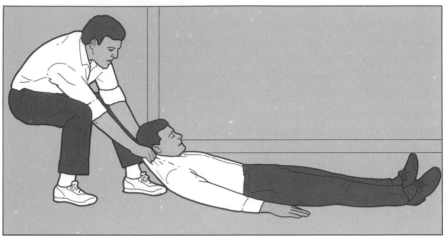

Figure 52
Clothes Drag

• If the victim is very large, you can use the foot drag *(Fig. 53)* as long as the victim's head will not be injured by bumpy or rough ground.

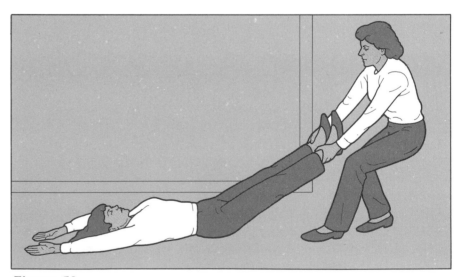

Figure 53
Foot Drag

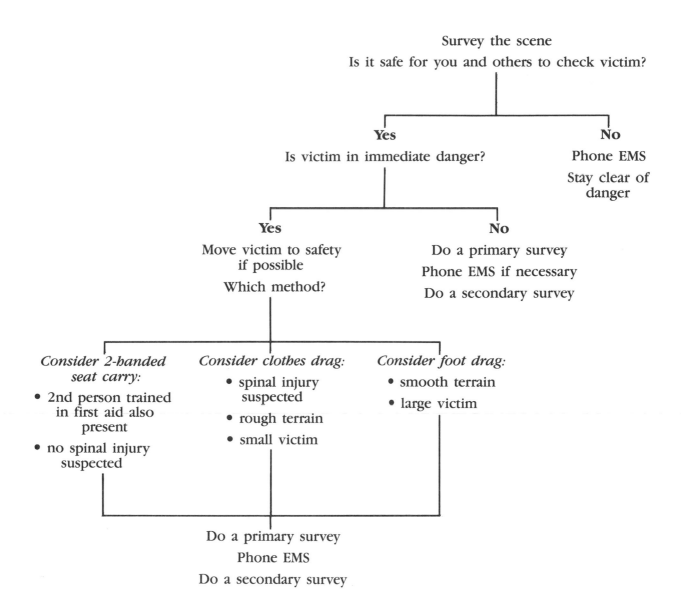

Survey the scene
Is it safe for you and others to check victim?

Yes
Is victim in immediate danger?

No
Phone EMS
Stay clear of danger

Yes
Move victim to safety if possible
Which method?

No
Do a primary survey
Phone EMS if necessary
Do a secondary survey

Consider 2-handed seat carry:
- 2nd person trained in first aid also present
- no spinal injury suspected

Consider clothes drag:
- spinal injury suspected
- rough terrain
- small victim

Consider foot drag:
- smooth terrain
- large victim

Do a primary survey
Phone EMS
Do a secondary survey

Appendix

The Emergency Medical Services (EMS) System

Throughout this course, you have learned how important it is for you and your community's EMS system to work together in order to give the victim of a medical emergency the best chance of survival.

This appendix explains what an EMS system is and how a victim of injury or sudden illness "enters" the system. It also explains the different types of care that a victim may require (basic life support and advanced life support) and what should happen when EMS personnel arrive at the scene of the emergency. At the end of this appendix there is a list of questions to help you learn more about your community's EMS system.

What Is an Emergency Medical Services (EMS) System?

To save a life in a life-threatening situation, two things must happen. Emergency care must be started right away by a trained bystander, and this care must be continued and enhanced by EMS personnel when they arrive. If no one with first aid training is nearby to begin emergency care immediately, or if the community's EMS system cannot quickly provide the right kind of help, then a victim's chances of survival may be greatly reduced.

By taking this course, you have already taken one step to improve the ability of your community's EMS system to save lives. You have increased the chances that a trained person—you—may be able to help at the scene of an accident or other medical emergency until EMS personnel arrive. Your ability to provide care immediately could save a life.

Components of an EMS system

Providing the victim with the right care at the right time is not an easy task. Although most communities have some way of sending medical help to victims of sudden illness or accidents, this help may not include everything that the victim needs and may not arrive in time to give the victim the best chance of surviving. Your community's ability to get the right help to the victim as quickly as possible requires both planning and resources. EMS systems that do this effectively usually have the following parts:

1. **Trained citizens** like you. Trained citizens can give first aid and alert the EMS system that a medical emergency has happened.

2. **Trained personnel.** To provide the best help quickly, an EMS system has specially trained personnel. These may include emergency medical technicians (EMTs), emergency medical technician-paramedics (paramedics), first responders (police, fire fighters), emergency dispatchers, and hospital emergency department physicians and nurses trained in emergency medicine.

3. **Special equipment.** Different situations and medical needs require specialized medical, rescue, and transportation equipment.

4. **Communications systems.** How well the EMS system works depends on how quickly citizens can alert the system that an emergency has happened, and how quickly the dispatcher can get the appropriate emergency personnel to the scene. Communications systems are also important because EMS personnel often need to communicate with the hospital emergency department as they care for the victim at the scene of the emergency and on the way to the hospital.

5. **Management and evaluation.** An EMS system needs a management structure which includes administration and coordination of all parts of the system, medical supervision and direction, and ongoing evaluation and research.

The Responsibilities of the Rescuer in the EMS System

In order for the victim of a medical emergency to receive care from the EMS system, the victim must enter the system. This means that the EMS system must be told about the emergency, and care should be given until EMS personnel arrive. These important first steps are generally performed by a citizen rescuer.

There are three things that you must do to make sure that a victim enters the EMS system with the best chance for survival:

1. **Recognize that a medical emergency has happened.** This isn't always easy. For example, you learned in Unit 4 that victims of heart attack often deny that they are having a heart attack, making it difficult for bystanders to know something is wrong. Also, victims of accidents may be so concerned about the well-being of another injured person that they may not realize that they themselves are hurt. Medical problems are not always obvious, but the skills you have learned in this course will help you recognize emergencies.

2. **Give first aid.** You have been trained to provide first aid for breathing, cardiac, and other emergencies. CPR, rescue breathing, and first aid for choking are all basic life support techniques. You have also learned to keep an injured person safe from further injury and as comfortable as possible until medical care can arrive.

3. Phone the EMS system for help. You may phone or direct bystanders to phone for help. Give all necessary information so that appropriate medical care can reach the scene of the emergency. This information is discussed in Unit 1.

How an EMS System Responds to a Call for Help

In many communities, a dispatcher will answer your call. The dispatcher is very important in making sure that the victim gets the right care immediately. In some systems, this person has special training to get specific information from the caller and to know which personnel and equipment to send to the scene. Some dispatchers can also give first aid instructions to the caller over the phone when it is necessary.

Basic Life Support and Advanced Life Support

As explained in Unit 1, the information you provide to the EMS dispatcher is important. It will help determine the type of care that the dispatcher sends to the scene of an emergency. The dispatcher may send either an ambulance capable of continuing basic life support, or an ambulance capable of delivering advanced life support. The care sent will depend on the needs of the victim and the services available in your community.

Most requests for emergency medical services require basic life support. For that reason, many states require that all ambulances be staffed with personnel trained to provide at least basic life support.

Some requests for assistance also require advanced life support. For example, a victim of heart attack or cardiac arrest requires both basic life support and advanced life support. Advanced life support personnel may be supervised by hospital-based physicians.

A key thing to remember is that basic life support and advanced life support must be given within specific time periods in order to give the victim the best chance of survival. That is why it is important to have a well-coordinated EMS system in your community. Highly trained personnel can do more to help the victim if they arrive promptly.

First Responder

When a dispatcher receives a call for emergency medical help the dispatcher will select the type of care that is needed and send the appropriate personnel. This may include police, fire, rescue, and ambulance personnel, depending on the type of emergency and the resources available at the time of the call.

In many communities, police and fire fighters may arrive at the scene before the ambulance because they are often located closer to the scene of the emergency. If you have been caring for a victim, the first responder may take over or ask you to assist. On the other hand, the first responder may tell you to continue care while he or she attends to other problems at the scene. It is important that you do not stop caring for a victim until the first responder takes over. You should expect the first responder to ask you for information about the victim. Information that you have gained from your primary and secondary surveys of the victim may be valuable to first responders, EMTs, paramedics, and to the hospital staff who will care for the victim later.

When the Ambulance Arrives
When the ambulance arrives, the EMTs or paramedics will take over responsibility for care of the victim and will provide additional medical care. Their goal is to begin to stabilize the victim's condition (correct life-threatening problems) at the scene. Once this has been done, the EMS personnel will prepare the victim for transport to the appropriate hospital emergency department, and they will continue caring for the victim on the way. When the ambulance arrives at the hospital, the EMS personnel will transfer responsibility for care of the victim to the emergency room staff.

You and Your EMS System

As you can see, the process by which you and the EMS system work together to save lives is complex. You should know that many communities do not have EMS systems that contain all of the features described above.

If you have ever been concerned about someone close to you having a heart attack or being the victim of a medical emergency, you owe it to yourself to find out what type of care your community's EMS system can provide in an emergency before an emergency happens. When minutes count, your knowledge of your community's EMS system can help you make the right decisions. The following checklist has been included to help you find out more about your community's EMS system.

Assessing Your Community's Emergency Medical Services (EMS) System

With a better idea of the different parts and responsibilities of a community emergency medical services system, you will be better able to assess the emergency medical services offered by your own community.

Your answers to the following questions will help you evaluate the services that your community provides. The questions to which you answer YES will show you the strengths of your community's EMS system. The questions to which you answer NO will point out areas where your community's EMS system could be strengthened. As a citizen and a taxpayer, your support of your community's EMS system is as important as your knowing how to perform first aid.

EMS Questionnaire

The following questions reflect the EMS standards set forth in the Emergency Medical Services Systems Act of 1973, the federal EMS legislation.

1. Are regularly scheduled CPR and first aid classes, open to the public, offered in your community? YES _____ NO _____

2. Does your community have a 9-1-1 emergency number for EMS, fire, and police? YES _____ NO _____

3. Do your local schools certify students in first aid and CPR? YES _____ NO _____

4. Are local police officers trained and certified in American Red Cross First Aid or in the U.S. Department of Transportation First Responder training? YES _____ NO _____

5. Is your local ambulance service staffed by EMTs? YES _____ NO _____

6. Does your local ambulance service regularly leave the station to answer an emergency call within two minutes of receiving the call? YES _____ NO _____

7. Does your community have advanced life support units staffed by EMT-paramedics? YES _____ NO _____

8. Are rescue services in your community (EMS, police, fire) provided by well-equipped units staffed by EMTs? YES _____ NO _____

9. Are all emergency services in your community dispatched and coordinated through a central emergency communications center? YES _____ NO _____

10. Is your nearest hospital emergency department staffed on a 24-hour basis by physicians and nurses who are specially trained in emergency medicine? YES _____ NO _____

11. Does your community have a plan to transfer very acutely ill or injured patients to specialty centers? YES _____ NO _____

12. Does your community have an area-wide disaster plan to deal with multi-casualty incidents, natural disasters, and environmental emergencies? YES _____ NO _____

13. Is there one office in charge of the administration, coordination, and evaluation of the EMS system? YES _____ NO _____

Adapted from "A Community Scoring Guide for Emergency Health Services," Office of Emergency Medical Services, The Pennsylvania State University.

Glossary

ABCs—*A*irway, *B*reathing, and *C*irculation, checked when doing a primary survey.

Abdominal Thrust—An upward push to the abdomen given to clear the airway of a person with a complete airway obstruction.

Abrasion—An open wound with damage to the skin from a scrape by a hard surface.

Action Guide—A part of each unit in this workbook that clearly and simply identifies the appropriate order of steps to take in caring for a specific first aid problem.

Adam's Apple—The protruding part in the front of the neck formed by the thyroid cartilage.

Air-Borne—Carried in or transmitted by air; certain diseases such as influenza are air-borne.

Air Exchange—The process of respiration or breathing; inhalation and exhalation of air into and out of the lungs.

Airway—The passageway through which air enters the body and goes to the lungs.

Airway Obstruction—Partial or complete blockage of the airway. See **anatomic obstruction** and **mechanical obstruction.**

Allergic Reaction—A reaction, sometimes severe, to certain substances such as the poison in insect bites and stings; may cause hives, severe swelling, redness, difficult breathing, loss of consciousness, or death.

Anatomic Obstruction—Blockage of the airway by the tongue or by tissues of the throat.

Apathy—A lack of interest or concern.

Arterial Bleeding—Bleeding from an artery, characterized by a bright red, spurting flow.

Arteries—The blood vessels that carry blood from the heart to the cells of the body.

Artificial Pulse—Cardiac pulse that is felt on a victim while chest compressions are being performed.

Artificial Respiration—See **rescue breathing.**

Avulsion—An injury in which a portion of the skin and sometimes other soft tissue is partly or completely torn from the body.

Bacteria—Microscopic organisms that can cause disease.

Blood-borne—Carried by the blood. Certain diseases such as hepatitis are blood-borne.

Blood Pressure—The force of the circulating blood pushing against walls of the blood vessels.

Blood Vessels—The tubes through which blood circulates throughout the body.

Brachial Artery—The artery that supplies blood to the arm.

Breastbone—The main bone in the front, center part of the chest to which the ribs are connected.

Breathlessness—The absence of breathing.

Capillaries—The smallest blood vessels.

Capillary Bleeding—Blood flow from the capillaries.

Cardiac Arrest—The condition when the heart stops beating; CPR must be given promptly to keep blood flowing to the brain and the cells of the body.

CPR—The abbreviation for **cardiopulmonary resuscitation.**

Cardiac Emergency—A life-threatening condition when the heart is not functioning properly, such as during a heart attack or a cardiac arrest.

Glossary

Cardiopulmonary Resuscitation—An emergency procedure for a person who is not breathing and whose heart has stopped beating (cardiac arrest). The procedure involves a combination of chest compressions and rescue breathing.

Cardiovascular Disease—A disease characterized by the gradual clogging of the blood vessels by fatty substances; associated with heart attack, stroke, high blood pressure, and diabetes.

Carotid Artery—The artery that supplies blood to the head.

Carotid Pulse—The beat that is felt at the side of the neck when the carotid artery is pressed. Located between the windpipe and the neck muscle, the carotid pulse is checked to determine the presence or absence of heartbeat. See **pulse.**

Chest Compression—A procedure for manually circulating blood in a person whose heart has stopped beating. It involves pressing up and down on the lower half of the breastbone. CPR is a combination of chest compressions and rescue breathing.

Chest Thrusts—Technique of pressing on the middle of the breastbone, used to clear the airway. Chest thrusts are used for an adult with a complete airway obstruction who is extremely overweight or in the late stages of pregnancy.

Cholesterol—A fatty substance that builds up on the walls of arteries. It is a major contributor to heart disease.

Circulatory Emergency—A life-threatening emergency in which the beat of the heart stops or is disrupted.

Circulatory System—The system that carries blood to all the cells in the body. Its components are blood, blood vessels, and the heart. Also known as the cardiovascular system.

Closed Fracture—A broken or cracked bone with no visible wound.

Complete Airway Obstruction—A condition in which a person is choking and unable to speak, cough, or breathe.

Cross Contamination—The transmission of a disease from one person to another through the blood infected with that disease.

Decontamination—A thorough cleansing to reduce germs and contaminants.

Diabetes—A condition caused by the inadequate production of the hormone insulin.

Diabetic Coma—A medical emergency in which a person with diabetes is seriously affected by the lack of insulin.

Emergency Action Principles—The four basic steps to be followed in all emergency situations to ensure that victims receive proper care.

EMS—The abbreviation for emergency medical services.

EMS Dispatcher—A member of the emergency medical services (EMS) system who receives emergency calls and directs the appropriate personnel and equipment to the scene of a medical emergency.

Emergency Medical Services (EMS) System—A community-based system that delivers specialized care for victims who are ill or injured. Care is provided at the scene of the emergency and is continued during transportation to and following arrival at an appropriately staffed and equipped health-care facility.

Femoral Artery—The artery that supplies blood to the leg.

Finger Sweep—A technique used as part of the procedure to dislodge and remove a piece of food or an object from the airway of an unconscious choking victim.

Foreign Body—An object that lodges in a person's airway, causing an obstruction or blockage of the airway.

Frostbite—An injury to body tissues caused by the formation of ice crystals in those tissues.

Gangrene—The death of an area of soft tissues due to a loss of the blood supply.

Germs—Disease-producing microorganisms.

Head-tilt/Chin-lift—A technique used to open the airway of an unconscious person. It is done by applying backward pressure to the forehead and lifting the jaw. This tilts the head back and lifts the chin.

Heart Attack—A condition in which blood flow to part of the heart is blocked, causing that part of the heart muscle to die from lack of oxygen.

Heat Cramps—Muscular pains and spasms resulting from loss of water and salt from the body.

Heat Exhaustion—A form of shock caused by heavy exercise or work in extreme heat.

Heat Stroke—A life-threatening condition in which the victim's temperature control system stops working.

Hypothermia—A general cooling of the body.

Implied Consent—A legal doctrine that applies to unconscious individuals, minors, mentally or emotionally disturbed, or badly injured or ill individuals who cannot respond. It assumes that if they could respond, they would consent to receiving emergency care.

Infectious Disease—A disease that may be transmitted or spread; a contagious disease.

Insulin Reaction—A diabetic emergency in which there is an excess of insulin in the blood causing low sugar levels.

Laceration—A cut, usually from a sharp object; may have jagged or smooth edges.

Manikin—A life-size model of a person, used for practicing first aid skills for respiratory and circulatory emergencies.

Mechanical Obstruction—Obstruction or blockage of the airway by a foreign object such as a piece of food.

Medical Alert Tag—A small tag, pendant, or container suspended from a necklace or bracelet; identifies the wearer as having a specific medical problem or condition and gives brief medical information.

Mouth-to-Mouth Breathing—A form of rescue breathing during which a person giving first aid breathes air into the mouth and lungs of a person who is not breathing.

Mouth-to-Nose Breathing—A form of rescue breathing in which a person giving first aid breathes air into the nose and lungs of a person who is not breathing. This is done when injuries or other difficulties make it impossible to perform mouth-to-mouth breathing.

Mouth-to-Stoma Breathing—A form of rescue breathing in which a person giving first aid breathes air into the stoma and lungs of a person who is not breathing.

Nausea—A feeling of sickness in the stomach with an urge to vomit.

9-1-1—A special telephone number used in many communities to give fast, direct connection to police, fire, and emergency medical services.

Notch—The place where the lower ribs meet the lower end of the breastbone in the center of the chest. Used as a reference point for finding the correct hand position for chest compressions.

Obstruction—Blockage. See **airway obstruction.**

Open Fracture—A broken or cracked bone with an open wound.

Oxygen—A gas that the cells of the body need in order to live. The air we breathe contains about 21 percent oxygen.

Oxygen-Rich Blood—Blood that contains oxygen.

Partial Airway Obstruction—A partial blockage of the airway that allows the victim to cough forcefully.

Poison Control Center—A center staffed by medical personnel who provide accurate information on how to care for victims of poisoning.

Pressure Point—A point where an artery runs near the bone and can be squeezed against that bone to reduce or control heavy bleeding.

Glossary

Primary Survey—A series of checks to discover conditions that are immediately life-threatening to a victim.

Pulmonary—Having to do with the lungs.

Pulse—The rhythmic "beat" in an artery. As the heart pumps blood, the walls of the artery expand and contract, causing a beat, or pulse. This beat, or pulse, can be felt by pressing on an artery.

Puncture—A small hole in the tissues with little external bleeding, caused by pointed objects.

Radial Pulse—The beat that is felt on the thumb side of the wrist. The radial pulse is checked to find out if the victim has a heartbeat.

Rescue Breathing—The process of breathing air into the lungs of a person who has stopped breathing. Also called **artificial respiration.**

Respiratory Emergency—A condition in which normal breathing is difficult or absent.

Respiratory System—The body system that draws air into the body and expels waste gases. The main parts are the airway and the lungs.

Risk Factors—Conditions and behaviors that increase the likelihood of a person's developing a disease. Some risk factors (age, sex, heredity) for cardiovascular disease cannot be changed. Others relate to lifestyle and can be changed.

Secondary Survey—A series of checks to discover conditions that are not immediately life-threatening to a victim but may become life-threatening if not corrected. These checks are done after life-threatening injuries have been found and cared for.

Seizure—A sudden attack, usually related to brain malfunction, that can be the result of diseased or injured brain tissue. More severe forms produce muscle contractions called convulsions.

Shock—The failure of the cardiovascular system to keep adequate oxygen-rich blood circulating to the vital organs of the body. Shock can be life-threatening.

Stoma—A surgically created opening in the front of the neck through which a person breathes.

Stroke—A condition in which one or more of the blood vessels to the brain become clogged or burst, causing a part of the brain to die from lack of oxygen.

Traumatic Injury—An injury caused by violence or force.

Universal Distress Signal—An action in which a choking victim grasps at his or her throat to signal that he or she is choking.

Unresponsiveness—A condition in which a person does not respond to verbal or physical stimuli.

Vein—A blood vessel that carries blood back to the heart.

Venous Bleeding—Loss of blood from a vein.

Vital Organs—Essential organs of the body, such as the heart, brain, and lungs.

Vital Signs—The signs of life: the pulse, breathing, and skin appearance (temperature, color, moisture).

Index

Index

Index

Index

Instructions for Emergency Phone Calls

Emergency Phone Numbers

EMS _____ Fire _____ Police _____

Doctor's name _____ Number _____

Poison Control Center _____

Other important numbers

    Name _____ Number _____

    Name _____ Number _____

    Name _____ Number _____

Name of medical facility with 24-hour emergency

care _____

Information for Emergency Call (Be prepared to give this information to the EMS dispatcher.)

1. Location

    Street address _____

    City or town _____

    Directions (cross streets, landmarks, etc.)

    _____

2. Phone number from which call is made _____

3. Caller's name _____

4. What happened _____

5. How many injured _____

6. Condition of victim(s) _____

7. Help (first aid) being given _____

Note: Do not hang up first. Let the person you called hang up first.

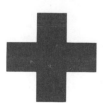

**American
Red Cross**

Notes

American Red Cross First Aid:
When an Adult Stops Breathing

1 **Does the Person Respond?**
- Tap or gently shake victim.
- Shout, "Are you OK?"

2 **Shout, "Help!"**
- Call people who can phone for help.

3 **Roll Person Onto Back**
- Roll victim toward you by pulling slowly.

4 **Open Airway**
- Tilt head back and lift chin.

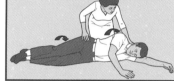

5 **Check for Breathing**
- Look, listen, and feel for breathing for 3 to 5 seconds.

6 **Give 2 Full Breaths**
- Keep head tilted back.
- Pinch nose shut.
- Seal your lips tight around victim's mouth.
- Give 2 full breaths for 1 to 1½ seconds each.

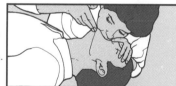

7 **Check for Pulse at Side of Neck**
- Feel for pulse for 5 to 10 seconds.

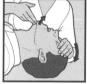

8 **Phone EMS for Help**
- Send someone to call an ambulance.

9 **Begin Rescue Breathing**
- Keep head tilted back.
- Lift chin.
- Pinch nose shut.
- Give 1 full breath every 5 seconds.
- Look, listen, and feel for breathing between breaths.

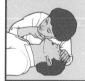

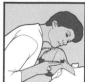

10 **Recheck Pulse Every Minute**
- Keep head tilted back.
- Feel for pulse for 5 to 10 seconds.
- If victim has pulse but is not breathing, continue rescue breathing. If no pulse, begin CPR.

American Red Cross

Local Emergency (EMS) Telephone Number: _____

Everyone should learn how to perform the steps above, how to give first aid for choking, and CPR. Call your local American Red Cross chapter _____ (chapter telephone number) for information on these techniques and other first aid courses.

Notes

American Red Cross First Aid:

When an Adult Is Choking

1 Ask, "Are You Choking?"

2 Shout, "Help!"

Call for help if victim—
- Cannot cough, speak, or breathe.
- Is coughing weakly.
- Is making high-pitched noises.

3 Phone EMS for Help
- Send someone to call an ambulance.

4 Do Abdominal Thrusts
- Wrap your arms around victim's waist.
- Make a fist.
- Place thumbside of fist on middle of victim's abdomen just above navel and well below lower tip of breastbone.
- Grasp fist with your other hand.
- Press fist into abdomen with a quick upward thrust.

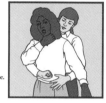

Repeat abdominal thrusts until object is coughed up, or victim starts to breathe or cough.

If victim becomes unconscious, lower victim to floor.

5 Do a Finger Sweep
- Grasp tongue and lower jaw and lift jaw.
- Slide finger down inside of cheek to base of tongue.
- Sweep object out.

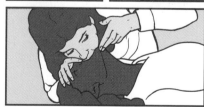

6 Open Airway
- Tilt head back and lift chin.

7 Give 2 Full Breaths
- Keep head tilted back.
- Pinch nose shut.
- Seal your lips tight around victim's mouth.
- Give 2 full breaths for 1 to 1½ seconds each.

8 Give 6 to 10 Abdominal Thrusts

If air won't go in—
- Place heel of one hand against middle of victim's abdomen.
- Place other hand on top of first hand.
- Press into abdomen with quick upward thrusts.

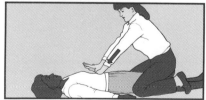

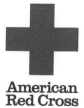

Repeat steps 5, 6, 7, and 8, until airway is cleared, or ambulance arrives.

Local Emergency (EMS) Telephone Number: _____

Everyone should learn how to perform the above steps and how to give rescue breathing and CPR. Call your local American Red Cross chapter _____ (chapter telephone number) for information on these techniques and other first aid courses. Caution: Abdominal thrusts (the Heimlich maneuver) may cause injury. Do not practice on a person.

American Red Cross

Notes

American Red Cross First Aid:
CPR for an Adult

1 *Does the Person Respond?*
- Tap or gently shake victim.
- Shout, "Are you OK?"

2 *Shout, "Help!"*
- Call people who can phone for help.

3 *Roll Person Onto Back*
- Roll victim toward you by pulling slowly.

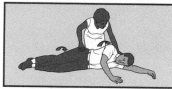

4 *Open Airway and Check for Breathing*
- Tilt head back and lift chin.
- Look, listen, and feel for breathing for 3 to 5 seconds.

5 *Give 2 Full Breaths*
- Keep head tilted back.
- Pinch nose shut.
- Seal your lips tight around victim's mouth.
- Give 2 full breaths for 1 to 1½ seconds each.

6 *Check for Pulse at Side of Neck*
- Feel for pulse for 5 to 10 seconds.

7 *Phone EMS for Help*
- Send someone to call an ambulance.

8 *Find Hand Position*
- Locate notch at lower end of breastbone.
- Place heel of other hand on breastbone, next to fingers.

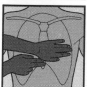

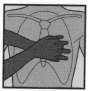

- Remove hand from notch and put it on top of other hand.
- Keep fingers off chest.

9 *Give 15 Compressions*
- Position shoulders over hands.
- Compress breastbone 1½ to 2 inches.
- Do 15 compressions in approximately 10 seconds.

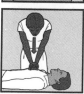

10 *Give 2 Full Breaths*
- Tilt head back and lift chin.
- Pinch nose shut.
- Seal your lips tight around victim's mouth.
- Give 2 full breaths for 1 to 1½ seconds each.

11 *Repeat Compression/ Breathing Cycles*
- Do 4 cycles of 15 compressions and 2 breaths.
- Recheck pulse after 1 minute. If no pulse, give 2 full breaths and continue CPR.

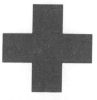

Local Emergency (EMS) Telephone Number: _____

Everyone should learn how to perform the steps above and how to give first aid for breathing and choking emergencies. Call your local American Red Cross chapter _____ (chapter telephone number) for information on these techniques and other first aid courses.

American Red Cross

Notes